KU-312-505

30 SECRETS OF THE WORLD'S HEALTHIEST CUISINES

Global Eating Tips and Recipes from China, France, Japan, the Mediterranean, Africa, and Scandinavia

Steven Jonas, M.D.
Sandra J. Gordon

LIBRARY
THE NORTH HIGHLAND COLLEGE
- 2 MAY 2000

John Wiley & Sons, Inc.
New York • Chichester • Weinheim • Brisbane • Singapore • Toronto

This book is printed on acid-free paper. ∞

Copyright © 2000 by Steven Jonas and Sandra J. Gordon. All rights reserved

Published by John Wiley & Sons, Inc.
Published simultaneously in Canada

Pie chart illustration on p. 119 by Jackie Aher

No part of this publication may be reproduced, stored in a retrieval system or transmitted in any form or by any means, electronic, mechanical, photocopying, recording, scanning or otherwise, except as permitted under Sections 107 or 108 of the 1976 United States Copyright Act, without either the prior written permission of the Publisher, or authorization through payment of the appropriate per-copy fee to the Copyright Clearance Center, 222 Rosewood Drive, Danvers, MA 01923, (978) 750-8400, fax (978) 750-4744. Requests to the Publisher for permission should be addressed to the Permissions Department, John Wiley & Sons, Inc., 605 Third Avenue, New York, NY 10158-0012, (212) 850-6011, fax (212) 850-6008, E-Mail: PERMREQ@WILEY.COM.

The information contained in this book is not intended to serve as a replacement for professional medical advice. Any use of the information in this book is at the reader's discretion. The author and the publisher specifically disclaim any and all liability arising directly or indirectly from the use or application of any information contained in this book. A health care professional should be consulted regarding your specific situation.

ISBN: 0471-35263-2

Printed in the United States of America

10 9 8 7 6 5 4 3 2 1

00329351
29351

30 Secrets of the
World's Healthiest Cuisines

LIBRARY

LIBRARY
THE NORTH HIGHLAND COLLEGE
- 2 MAY 2000

For my mom, Florence Kyzor Jonas,
for whom this book is especially meaningful.

—S.J.

For my husband, Ron Agababian,
an exemplary global eater,
and my parents,
Sharon J. and Frederick J. Gordon,
from whom I learned the value
of sustained effort.

—S.J.G.

29351

641.563 JON

LIBRARY
THE NORTH HIGHLAND COLLEGE

− 2 MAY 2000

Contents

Acknowledgments

Special thanks to all those near and far who agreed to be interviewed for this book and, thus, made it possible. We are also grateful to our literary agent, Linda Konner, for her sage advice and unflagging support.

Making Your Diet Go Global

Like wearing your seat belt and driving at safe speeds, adopting better food and health habits can improve your chances of dying young, late in life. For example:

- The American Cancer Society estimates that one-third of all cancer deaths in the United States are related to nutrition. According to the American Institute for Cancer Research, a nonprofit educational organization based in Washington, D.C., eating right coupled with not smoking have the potential to reduce your cancer risk by 60 to 70 percent.

- According to the American Heart Association, a balanced low-fat diet can help you beat heart disease by reducing one of the major risk factors for heart attack—high blood cholesterol—as well as high blood pressure.

- Your diet and your fitness routine can help you guard against weight gain to minimize, delay, or possibly even prevent Type 2 (non-insulin-dependent) diabetes and osteoarthritis, the condition in which the cartilage around joints and adjacent bones gradually deteriorates.

- Your eating habits can help you maintain optimal bone health and prevent age-related bone loss. By eating right, you're less likely to become one of the growing number of frail elderly.

- What you eat can even affect, in general, how well you age. Many gerontologists are now investigating the scientific evidence concerning the influence of lifestyle factors on aging. As a result, they're stressing that your daily habits, including your diet, can actually shape underlying genetic tendencies to increase your *health*span, that is, the years of your life when you truly feel vibrant, vital, and healthy.

But what should you eat to stay healthy? The U.S. Department of Agriculture (USDA) periodically issues dietary guidelines for Americans to show them how to get adequate energy and nutrients while minimizing the risk for chronic disease. According to the latest guidelines, you're on the right track if you:

1 Eat a variety of foods.
2 Balance the food you eat with physical activity; maintain or improve your weight.
3 Choose a diet with plenty of grain products, vegetables, and fruits.
4 Choose a diet low in fat, saturated fat, and cholesterol.
5 Choose a diet moderate in sugars.
6 Choose a diet moderate in salt and sodium.
7 Drink alcoholic beverages only in moderation.

In conjunction with the dietary guidelines, the USDA designed the Food Guide Pyramid to help you visualize just how many servings of food from each food group constitutes a healthy diet.

Trouble is, meeting the goals of the dietary guidelines and the Food Guide Pyramid with the standard North American diet can sometimes mean repeating the same old meals, leaving you hungry for a more interesting approach. Without diverging from these sensible ground rules, you could try a new variation on the theme of using your diet to maximize your health—one that's more colorful, more flavorful, and *more motivating.* Venture off the well-worn path of the typical North American diet and model your eating and lifestyle habits after those found in the countries that report the lowest rates of major diseases. In short, make your diet go global. Let the best eating habits of the world's healthiest countries inspire you. That is what this book is about, and what is hoped that reading it will do for you.

Why Global Eating?

From politics to the environment, there's a global emphasis on just about everything these days—and healthy eating is no exception. From across the

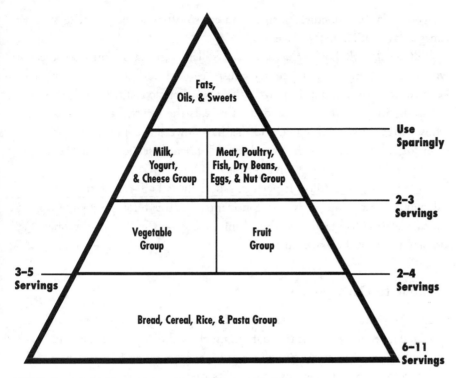

Fats,
Oils, & Sweets

Milk,
Yogurt,
& Cheese Group

Meat, Poultry,
Fish, Dry Beans,
Eggs, & Nut Group

Use
Sparingly

Vegetable
Group

Fruit
Group

2–3
Servings

3–5
Servings

2–4
Servings

Bread, Cereal, Rice, & Pasta Group

6–11
Servings

USDA's Food Guide Pyramid: A guide to daily food choices.

Atlantic and the Pacific Oceans come important nutrition research and data. To improve our health, international research suggests we may benefit by importing the best eating habits from countries that report comparatively low rates of nutrition-related disease.

From fiber in Finland to red wine in France, nutrition studies have gone global. But what does it all mean to North Americans? Can we glean anything from France, for example, where the average person gets a greater percentage of calories from fat than his or her American counterpart, but is much less likely to develop heart disease? Can we gather anything from Japan, where the average life expectancy is the highest in the world? Can we take away anything from China, where cancer rates are remarkably low? The answer is yes.

By incorporating the diet secrets from around the world discussed throughout this book, you may lower your chances of developing a number of major diet-related diseases such as cancer, heart disease, diabetes, osteoarthritis, and osteoporosis. Granted, your diet is only one part of the total equation for good health. Nonetheless, since you eat so often—perhaps at least three times a day—it's a major player.

30 Secrets of the World's Healthiest Cuisines blends the latest nutrition research with information about the culinary histories and traditions of a number of key countries from around the world to provide practical tips to increase the disease-fighting power of your diet. It reveals the health habits of countries whose citizens live the longest, and that have lower incidences and death rates of major chronic diseases than we do. You'll learn their diet secrets for staying healthy and for getting and staying slim.

Of course, no country is perfect, especially as U.S.-style fast-food establishments set up shop across the continents. But this book points the way to which *traditional* habits are worthy of importing—as well as to the ones that are better left on their own turf.

A Guide to Daily Food Choices

Chapter 2 ventures south to reveal the healthy eating secrets of the Mediterranean. The eating patterns throughout much of this region conform to six of the seven USDA dietary guidelines, and have done so for centuries. The Mediterranean region demonstrates by its desirable health statistics that not all fat is the enemy—that it's the kind and amount of fat in your diet that matters.

Chapter 3 discusses the Chinese diet—how the Chinese who live in China report lower rates of cancer and diabetes than do North Americans, and how they manage to consume an average of 300 more calories a day per person than do North Americans without worrying about obesity. You'll discover how the Chinese manage to follow a diet that naturally conforms to six of the seven USDA dietary guidelines.

Chapter 4 travels to France to study the French Paradox. You'll learn the healthy eating secrets of a country ironically famed for rich sauces, triple-fat cheeses, duck-liver pâté, and chocolate mousse—a clear violation of USDA dietary guideline number four: Choose a diet low in fat, saturated fat, and cholesterol. Yet, you'll learn how the French have less heart disease than North Americans. Chapter 4 also divulges the dietary factors that enable the French to maintain a healthy weight and keep their enviable figures.

Chapter 5 explains how the Japanese diet can potentially help you reduce your risk of cancer and heart disease and maximize longevity. The Japanese have comparatively low rates of cancer and heart disease as well as the world's lengthiest life expectancy. Chapter 5 also provides insight into the tricks the Japanese use to maintain a healthy weight and to follow a diet that's low in fat, saturated fat, and cholesterol without getting bored.

Chapter 6 travels to certain parts of Scandinavia, where a high-fiber diet (USDA dietary guideline number three), among other factors, is thought to help people fight the battle against cancer and heart disease.

Chapter 7 explores the diet of the west coast of Africa—one rich in complex carbohydrates and a wealth of vegetables and grains. Perhaps it's no coincidence that breast cancer rates there are even lower than in Japan. No doubt, the diet is a contributing factor.

Building on these healthy cuisines from around the world, chapter 8 presents a menu plan you can use to truly transform and globalize your eating habits.

To help you easily follow the recommendations of chapter 8, chapter 9 gives you some ground rules and chapter 10 offers healthy recipes from the Global Kitchen, provided by renowned cooking school professionals and chefs from around the world. You'll learn how to import the eating habits of other countries by starting right in your own kitchen.

You Can Do It

Of course, if you've ever tried to modify your diet, you know that changing your eating and health habits is not easy. Eating habits, after all, are like old friends. They feel comfortable and familiar. But little by little, you can change them here and there to make a health difference. After all, many North Americans have already stopped smoking. According to a study by the National Cancer Institute, we're also eating more fruits, vegetables, and grain foods; between 1970 and 1994, per capita consumption of fruits rose by 22 percent; vegetables, by 19 percent; and grain products, by nearly 50 percent. (To learn more about the North American diet past and present, see the Appendix.) Similarly, *you* can take control of your eating habits—and of your health. This book gives you the road map you need. All that's required is a willingness to explore and a culinary sense of adventure.

THE MEDITERRANEAN

Olive Oil and Longevity

He is a shepherd or small farmer, a beekeeper or fisherman, or a tender of olives or vines. He walks to work daily and labors in the soft light of his Greek isle.... His midday, main meal is of eggplant, with large livery mushrooms, crisp vegetables and country bread dipped in the nectar that is golden Cretan olive oil. Once a week, there is a bit of lamb, naturally spiced from sheep grazing in thyme-filled pastures.

—Henry Blackburn, M.D., of the University of Minnesota Division of Epidemiology, describing the "real low-risk coronary male" documented to live on the Greek island of Crete.

Like the French Paradox, much has been written about the Mediterranean diet, the traditional diet circa 1960 of the olive-growing countries adjacent to the Mediterranean Sea, which has been evolving for centuries. Although there is no one Mediterranean diet, the diets of southern France, Italy, Spain, and Greece share several common denominators that make this healthful diet what it is. Its characteristics include an emphasis on fruits and vegetables as well as bread and grains such as bulgur, pasta, rice, couscous, and polenta. Fish, beans and other legumes, and nuts also figure prominently; cheese, yogurt, and other dairy products play supporting roles. Meat is only a small part of the diet. In the Mediterranean approach to eating, lean red meat is usually part of a meal only a few times a month. Those who can afford it, however, may occasionally eat meat more often, although almost always in humble quantities compared to North American standards.

The "Healthy Fat" Diet

One of the biggest hallmarks of the Mediterranean diet is its liberal use of olives and olive oil. As you may know, in this corner of the world, the diet is far from fat free. For centuries, the people of the Mediterranean have cooked with generous measures of the thick, emerald-gold, pungently flavored oil pressed from olives possibly harvested from trees growing right in their own backyard. Instead of using margarine or butter, they've cooked with olive oil, dipped their daily bread into pools of it, dressed their salads with it, and topped off prepared dishes with it, elevating olive oil to the principal role of garnish. Legend has it that the Greeks, in particular, even drank cupfuls of olive oil for breakfast before heading out to work in the fields.

"Indeed, in the Mediterranean region, there has always been a strong, albeit undocumented, belief that olive oil is the elixir of youth and health. Although one cannot take at face case reports or so-called popular wisdom, it's nevertheless intriguing that most centenarians in the Mediterranean have been inclined to attribute their longevity to diet in general and to olive oil and wine—two key ingredients in the Mediterranean diet—consumption in particular," writes Antonia Trichopoulou, M.D., and Pagona Lagiou, M.D., researchers with the National School of Public Health in Athens.

As you might expect, a significant percentage of the calories in the traditional Mediterranean diet comes from fat—around 30 percent in Italy to an excess of 42 percent on the Greek island of Crete. Yet, historically, the rates of heart disease in Mediterranean countries have been as much as 90 percent lower than the rates in the United States, as if fat and heart disease weren't related.

We'll Have What They're Having

How do they do it? Back in the 1950s and 1960s, when scientific interest in the Mediterranean diet was first ignited, nutrition researchers began asking that very question. At the time, while the people of the Mediterranean were dining on fish they may have actually caught themselves, dousing home-grown vegetables and grain-based salads with olive oil, and washing it all down with a glass of wine, scores of North Americans were marveling over their TV dinners, thanks to the introduction of the home freezer. We were also flocking to local drive-in eateries. Hundreds of fast-food restaurants were popping up across the country. Steak, juicy and fatty, was often the main attraction at dinner two and three times a week for many typical middle-class families.

It's no surprise then, that many North Americans of the 1960s got 45 percent of their total daily calories from fat, much of it saturated (about 11 percent more fat than consumed, on average, in 1995). Thousands of middle-aged executives in North America (and in northern Europe, where the diet was equally dense in saturated fat) were dropping dead from heart attacks at an increasingly alarming rate. Could it be because of their diet? Back then, a relationship between diet and heart disease was a novel notion.

Fat Finding

To investigate the possible relationship between fat and heart disease, renowned researcher Ansel Keyes conducted the Seven Countries study, a ground-breaking international research initiative that put to the test the diets of over twelve thousand men in rural areas of Yugoslavia, Finland, Italy, the Netherlands, Greece, the United States, and Japan. From 1958 to 1964, these men—ages forty to fifty-nine—were poked and prodded and asked detailed questions about their health habits and their daily diet.

The Seven Countries study, one of the first to make the connection between heart disease and dietary fat, concluded that the type of fat consumed in the diet was more important for good health than was the total amount of fat.

Although initially rebuffed by selected committees of cardiologists, the study's conclusions were an "aha" for those who were ready to accept it. It introduced the now widely accepted theory that the populations who consumed the most saturated fat had the highest blood serum cholesterol levels and the greatest incidences of heart attack.

The Mediterranean Diet Now

Unfortunately, as with many of the traditional diets the world over, the traditional diet throughout much of the Mediterranean is slowly fading, especially in urban areas. Yes, they're still using olive oil, often the highly regarded extra-virgin kind, which is what Dr. Trichopoulou calls "olive fruit juice." Less acidic than those labeled "virgin" or "pure," extra-virgin olive oil is replete with vitamin E and perhaps other disease-fighting antioxidants that have yet to be discovered. But as a result of higher income and advances in refrigerated transportation throughout the Mediterranean, butter and margarine, with their harmful saturated and partially hydrogenated trans fatty acids (manufactured fat), and polyunsaturated fats like corn oil are creeping into the diet in most areas. Meat is also gaining staple status. Imported meats in Greece, for example, have increased more than fourfold from 1975 to 1985. Referring specifically to urban Greeks, "They're in danger," concludes Dorothea Klimis, Ph.D., a

---

A Note from Dr. Jonas
WE'VE COME A LONG WAY

Americans got 45 percent of their calories from fat in 1965. By 1995, thanks to public health campaigns and the bad press that saturated fat has received, the numbers were down to 34 percent. But before you pat yourself on the back, take note: Total fat consumption appears to be slowly on the rise, in sync with total calorie intake. It's right to eat less fat, but to make a health difference, you also need to consume fewer calories.

native of Greece and a professor of food science and human nutrition at the University of Maine, who has studied the dietary habits of Greece as part of a multinational project known as the European Prospective Investigation into Cancer and Nutrition (EPIC).

Indeed, en route to the Parthenon or the Acropolis from central Athens, you're likely to pass dozens of restaurants and local establishments serving North American–style sandwiches such as grilled cheese with ham, a sight that makes epidemiologists shudder. Granted, you'll also see many locals carrying bags of fruit. But in retail kiosks throughout Greece, you'll notice Pringles potato chips for sale—just one example of the kinds of U.S. products that were unavailable even five years ago. Consequently, according to studies, the present Mediterranean diet is heftier than ever—for example, in urban Greece, close to a shocking 50 percent of total calories are coming from fat. The diet is now similar to what the North American diet was back in 1965, when our awareness of diet's link to disease was in its infancy.

Meanwhile, smoking continues to be widespread throughout the Mediterranean. And with massive urbanization, the live-off-the-land kinds of exercise that were once everyday components of the lifestyle for many— shepherding, farming, fishing, and beekeeping—have become a thing of the past. Speaking of the Greeks in Mediterranean urban areas, Dr. Trichopoulou says, "They don't walk anymore and they don't exercise. We are lazy." Consequently, Mediterranean-based researchers like Dr. Trichopoulou fear the advent of a dramatic change in heart disease statistics in the near future as the sedentary, high-fat lifestyle manifests itself on patient medical charts.

Healthy Traditions

The good news? Although the traditional Mediterranean diet is now succumbing to North American influences, disease statistics and incidence rates show that centuries of eating the Mediterranean way are still on the side of the people of the region. American Heart Association statistics from 1992 to 1995, for example, indicate that Spain, Italy, Greece, and France still report significantly lower death rates from cardiovascular disease than does the United States. Each of these countries also shows only a fraction of the U.S. incidence rates for breast, prostate, lung, and colon cancer—four major health threats in North America. Furthermore, on average, the people of the Mediterranean still live about a year longer than U.S. citizens.

Clearly, the Mediterranean diet hasn't completely morphed into the North American–style diet yet. But this chapter focuses mainly on the traditional, rather than the transitional, Mediterranean diet—the one enjoyed up to about 1960, before large-scale trade and rising incomes began effecting change. How did the people of the Mediterranean resist heart disease and other conditions while consuming the traditional high-fat diet? How can you benefit? This chapter shows you how making just a few Mediterranean-inspired diet changes can help you increase the health-promoting potential of your diet and perhaps even grant you a life that's longer, healthier, and less stressed.

Food for Thought

What country today has the best diet? When asked that question in a 1997 Eating Well article, Ansel Keyes, also known as "the father of modern nutrition," replied: "I'd say the healthiest diet in the world is found in rural parts of southern Italy, around the Mediterranean." He should know. Keyes, now in his mid-nineties, has lived in that region for decades.

The Traditional Mediterranean Diet at a Glance

Rich in "healthy" fats, including olive oil and omega-3 fatty acids

- The traditional diet, which is rich in olive oil, gets 30 to 42 percent of its calories from fat, yet the people who consumed it regularly reported significantly low rates of cancer and heart disease, suggesting that dietary fat isn't necessarily the enemy. It's the type of fat, not the amount of fat, that matters.

- Omega-3 fatty acids from fish and wild greens, such as purslane, also play an important role.

Vegetables abound; meat is minor

- Meat takes a backseat to fruits and vegetables, legumes and grains, and is perhaps another factor behind the comparatively low rates of heart disease and cancer.

Loads of beneficial herbs

- Many of the herbs traditionally used to flavor Mediterranean foods—such as rosemary and parsley—are believed to contain cancer-fighting antioxidants.

Moderate drinking

- Traditional Mediterranean people are also temperate wine drinkers. Moderate alcohol consumption, as echoed by the French Paradox, has been associated with a reduced risk of heart disease and other maladies.

Slower pace of life contributes to the diet's healthfulness

- The Mediterranean diet is more than a diet. It's a lifestyle marked by a leisurely pace and a strong sense of social connection, which may also contribute to the reduced risk of disease in this part of the world.

Food for Thought

Spaniards live longer than most other nationalities. According to the Statistics Office of the European Community, life expectancy in Spain is the second highest in the world, after Japan. In 1998, mean life expectancy in Spain was 78.2 years for men and 81.1 years for women, which is more than double their life expectancy in 1900.

The Fight against Cancer

The Mediterranean diet doesn't *just* protect you from heart disease. As the chart on page 13 shows, the incidence rates for all forms of cancer for men and women living in France, Spain, Italy, and Greece are, in some cases, nearly 50 percent less than the rates for U.S. residents.

GLOBAL EATING SECRET #1

Change Your Diet's Fat Mix

The traditional Mediterranean diet has always been high in heart-healthy monounsaturated fat found in the olive oil that the people have historically cooked with and dipped their pitas and baguettes into. Why is a diet that features olive oil healthier than, say, one that uses butter or corn oil? The secret is in olive oil's beneficial molecular structure. In essence, studies show that when you substitute foods high in monounsaturated fat—such as olive oil, canola oil, and almonds—for foods rich in saturated fat, such as red meat, poultry, butter, cheese, eggs, milk, and cream, you typically lower the unhealthy LDL cholesterol in your blood and raise healthy HDL cholesterol to reduce your risk of heart disease.

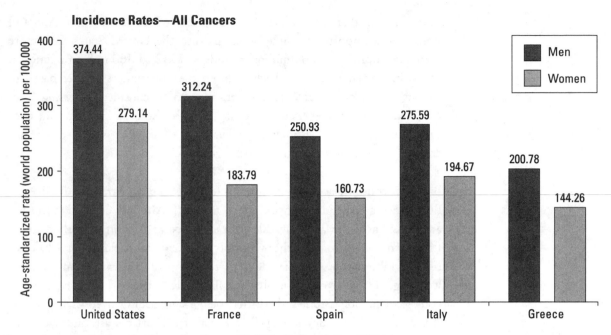

Incidence Rates—All Cancers

Source: *Inernational Agency for Research on Cancer, World Health Organization, 1990.*

The Health Benefits of Olive Oil

In further support of the benefits of olive oil, recent research suggests that it may also help fend off heart disease and cancer. Studies show that extra-virgin olive oil, for example, contains a high concentration of antioxidants called phenolic compounds that "scavenge" the free radicals in the blood. These free radicals can set the stage for the cell changes that lead to both heart disease and cancer. Moreover, studies show that women who consume diets high in monounsaturated fats like olive oil have a reduced risk of breast cancer. (The jury's still out, however, on olive oil's exact relationship to a reduced breast cancer risk; the lower risk may be due to mechanisms unrelated to monounsaturated fat.)

Perhaps as a result of all the good health reports about the Mediterranean diet presented by the media, Americans are consuming significantly

A Note from Dr. Jonas
THE PROBLEM WITH CORN OIL

Corn oil, a type of fat that seriously competes for Americans' food dollars, is predominantly polyunsaturated. That is, it's a type of fat that has been shown to lower LDL (bad) cholesterol. Trouble is, it also reduces HDL (good) cholesterol, so it's not as heart healthy as it might seem.

more olive oil than ever before. According to the North American Olive Oil Association, imports of edible olive oils into the United States have more than quadrupled, from 64 million pounds in 1992 to 360 million pounds in 1997. However, when Dr. Trichopoulou, the nutrition researcher based in Athens, was asked what North Americans should consider importing from the Mediterranean diet to improve their health, she didn't recommend consuming more olive oil. Rather, she advised, "I think what is needed is to increase the consumption of fruits and vegetables."

Based on consumption patterns, we're clearly on the right track with olive oil. But it's not a good idea to overdose on the stuff. After all, olive oil is still fat, and thus has twice as many calories per ounce as protein or carbohydrate. Like corn, safflower, and other vegetable oils, olive oil packs about 120 calories per tablespoon, so a diet doused with olive oil can easily contribute to weight gain, which can ultimately be harmful regardless of the type of fat you're consuming. Studies show that being significantly overweight can increase your odds of developing Type 2 diabetes, heart disease, and hypertension as well as cancers of the lung, colon/rectum, breast, and prostate.

If you're eating foods that contain fat, it's better to stick with healthier types of fat. Monounsaturated fats like olive and canola oils can change the fat chemistry of your blood to reduce your risk of heart disease and possibly cancer. Nonetheless, it's still a good idea to keep the total amount of fat in your diet at 30 percent or less of total calories, no more than 10 percent of which should come from saturated fat. If you've already switched from corn oil to olive or canola oil, good for you. Just be sure to substitute it for (not add it to) the saturated and polyunsaturated fats in your diet. Here are two quick practical tips you can use:

- When sautéing, use just enough olive or canola oil—instead of butter, corn, or safflower oil—to barely coat the bottom of the pan. Or skip the fat altogether, and sauté with nonfat chicken broth, vegetable broth, or nonfat cooking spray instead.

- When making salad dressing, drizzle in just a tablespoon or two of the finest extra-virgin olive oil, which packs the most flavor per calorie.

Are You Fat Phobic?

- Do you try to only eat foods labeled "low fat" or "nonfat"?

- Do you tend to eat the same foods over and over again because you know they're low in fat—for example, pasta with tomato sauce, plain bagels, and salad without dressing?

If you've answered yes to either of these questions, you could be seriously undermining the nutrition content of your diet. Skinning your chicken is a positive way to sensibly reduce the saturated fat in your diet, but you shouldn't be avoiding fat at all costs. After all, as the traditional Mediterranean diet has demonstrated, some fat can be good for you. And in fact, like a car, your body needs oil to run. Consider the health benefits of fat:

- On cold days, it's fat that keeps your body warm.
- Throughout your body, fat pads serve as shock absorbers, cushioning vital organs.
- Hormones are produced with fat, and your nervous system depends on fat to function properly.
- Fat nourishes every cell and helps your body absorb certain nutrients.
- When you dance all night or go for a long run, it's fat, specifically in a form called triglycerides (and a stored form of carbohydrates called glycogen), that fuels your performance.

Moreover, if you don't eat enough fat, your body will make its own saturated fat. Though this isn't a big problem in the United States, a diet that is exceptionally low in fat can turn the body into a very efficient fat-making machine.

Beware of Trans Fats

In addition to substituting olive and canola oils for the saturated fat in your diet, it makes sense to cut down on your diet's quotient of partially hydrogenated trans fatty acids. This type of fat—the manufactured fat found prominently in foods like stick margarine—is considered to be as unhealthy for your heart as is saturated fat.

"The traditional Mediterranean diet had zero partially hydrogenated trans fatty acids," says Walter Willet, M.D., professor of nutrition and epi-

---

A Note from Dr. Jonas
WHAT "NO MORE THAN 30 PERCENT OF A FOOD'S CALORIES SHOULD COME FROM FAT" REALLY MEANS

The actual guideline is: Total fat intake should provide no more than 30 percent of total calories. This applies to your *total* fat intake *over a week,* not to any one food, which is why there truly is room in your diet for a variety of foods—even high-fat ones, occasionally.

Food for Thought

Sicily is one area of the Mediterranean that has been virtually untouched by U.S. fast-food influences. What do Sicilians eat when they want a quick bite? Arancini *(balls of rice stuffed with prosciutto and mozzarella with Bolognese sauce),* pizza, calzone, or panelle *(chickpea fritters)*—all from local cafés, says Sara Schwartz, the co-proprietor of Tasting Places, www.tastingplaces.com, a cooking school that offers weeklong cooking classes in Sicily as well as other locations throughout Italy.

Food for Thought

Olives and olive oil contain not only healthy monounsaturated fat but also a phytochemical called squalene. Preliminary cancer studies show that squalene can battle the onset of lung, pancreatic, and breast cancers by inhibiting tumor formation.

Food for Thought

Forget about fat-free Olestra potato chips and sinless North American—style fat-free and low-fat brownies, cakes, cookies, and ice creams that crowd supermarket shelves. Naturally fat-free and low-fat foods have been popular in the Mediterranean for centuries. You'll find them at the street markets that display a rainbow section of fresh fruits and vegetables.

demiology at the Harvard School of Public Health. On the other hand, the American diet today is loaded with partially hydrogenated trans fatty acids, which are formed through the manufacturing process called hydrogenation, in which vegetable oil is hardened to become margarine or shortening.

The ingredients label on food products won't mention partially hydrogenated trans fats because they aren't yet regulated on food labels. But you can be sure that trans fats are lurking in shortening, processed pastries, cookies and crackers, french fries and other deep-fried fast foods, and of course, stick margarine. Studies have shown that partially hydrogenated trans fatty acids raise total cholesterol and LDL (bad) cholesterol. In very high amounts, trans fatty acids may even lower HDL (good) cholesterol. To eradicate much of this "bad" fat from your diet:

- Eat fewer processed snacks and deep-fried fast foods.

- Watch what you spread on your bread and toast. Instead of regular margarine (or butter, for that matter), use a diet margarine or a very soft tub margarine. In general, the harder the margarine or shortening, the more trans fats it contains. Or try almond butter (available at health food and grocery stores), which, like olive oil, is high in monounsaturated fat. Or just spread on jam.

GLOBAL EATING SECRET #2

Up Your Quota of Omega-3s

The Mediterranean diet contains another healthy fat that can help reduce your risk of disease: omega-3 fatty acids ("omega-3s"). People eating a traditional diet got omega-3 fatty acids from the fresh fish they caught from the Mediterranean Sea.

In addition, a regional delicacy called *chorta* (pronounced "hore-ta"), a blend of purslane and other wild greens, is an excellent Mediterranean omega-3 dietary source. Greece has over a hundred varieties of wild greens that grow in the hills, free for the picking and the eating, which make them especially appealing to rural peasants even today. Imagine gathering up the dandelions and other nuisance plants in your yard, steaming them, topping them off with extra-virgin olive oil and vinegar, and serving them for dinner. That's akin to what Greeks have been doing for centuries. And not only is *chorta* delicious, it's also good for you. "We have been surprised about the amount of flavonoids [disease-fighting phytochemicals] and the vitamins and minerals it contains," says Dr. Trichopolou.

Chorta also contains omega-3s. Purslane, a green commonly found in *chorta*, grows wild in the United States as well as in Greece. Maybe you've spotted this fleshy leafed plant with its pale yellow flowers and smooth, thick, reddish stems in your garden and tossed it into your compost pile. To Americans, purslane is an ignoble weed. But to the Greeks, it's a delicious delicacy that just happens to be packed with omega-3 fatty acids (its iron content is exceptionally high, too).

Omega-3s—The Underrated Fat

Omega-3 fatty acids are essential fatty acids (EFA) that your body needs to function. You must get EFAs from food because your body can't make them on its own. EFAs nourish every one of your cells and help regulate your hormones and keep your nervous system humming.

A wealth of research also shows that omega-3s protect against heart disease and reduce the risk of someone with heart disease dying of a heart attack. In one landmark study that dramatically demonstrated this point, 302 heart attack survivors were assigned to a slightly modified version of the traditional Mediterranean diet of the Greek island of Crete, which supplied 35 percent of its calories from fat. High in omega-3 fatty acids, this version of the Mediterranean diet featured fruits, vegetables, bread, whole grains, legumes, fish, olive oil, and moderate amounts of red wine, as well as a specially formulated omega-3–rich margarine (to pinch-hit for purslane). Another group of 303 heart attack patients were assigned a low-fat, "prudent," heart-healthy diet as recommended by the American Heart Association (AHA), which contained fewer fruits and vegetables and more beef, lamb, and pork. Only 30 percent of the calories in the prudent diet came from fat.

Although you'd think those on the prudent, heart-healthy diet would have won this round, the opposite proved true: Patients on the Mediterranean diet had an unprecedented 70 percent lower risk of dying from cardiovascular disease or of suffering from heart failure, heart attack, or stroke.

Subsequent news from the nutrition front indicates that there's even more to the omega-3 story. Besides helping fight heart disease, a diet rich in omega-3 may also detoxify harmful cancer-promoting enzymes in the lungs and other parts of the body. A four-year follow-up study involving 605 heart attack patients investigated the link between cancer risk and the traditional Mediterranean diet on the one hand, and the AHA heart-healthy diet on the other. According to the study, those on the Mediterranean diet were less likely to develop cancer than were the patients on the AHA diet. Researchers attributed their findings to the diet's ample amounts of fiber and antioxidants, such as the vitamin C in fruits and vegetables. They also credited the fact that those on the Mediterranean diet got more omega-3 fats and fewer omega-6 fats, a nonessential polyunsaturated fatty acid commonly found in vegetable oils such as corn, safflower, cottonseed, and sunflower. Just exactly how omega-3 fatty acids fight heart disease and cancer, however, is still being debated by the nutrition and medical community.

> **A Note from Dr. Jonas**
> BRAIN FOOD
>
> Docosahexaenoic acid (DHA), a type of fat in the omega-3 family, helps your brain function. In fact, a significant part of your brain is made from it. A diet high in omega-3 has been linked to the reduced risk of depression and Alzheimer's disease, as well as to enhanced intellectual performance. Moreover, breast milk contains both DHA and eicosapentaenoic acid (EPA), another fat in the omega-3 clan. Both DHA and EPA are important for infant brain development, which is another reason for the popular pro-breast-feeding expression "Breast is best."

Finding a Favorable Fat Ratio

The not-so-great news? The typical American diet tends to be low in omega-3 fatty acids and high in omega-6 fatty acids. Both omega-3 and omega-6 produce eicosanoids, hormonelike compounds in the body that regulate blood pressure, blood clotting, and other body functions. But studies show that the omega-6 eicosanoids can work against the benefits of omega-3 eicosanoids. The monounsaturated fat found in foods like olive oil and canola oil, however, doesn't have this blocking effect.

Some researchers conclude that the body functions best when the diet contains omega-6 and omega-3 fats in a ratio of about 4 to 1. (It's estimated that the current ratio of omega-6 to omega-3 fatty acids in the American diet is now more like 16 to 1.) The omega-6/omega-3 fat imbalance in the American diet has been linked to a number of serious illnesses and conditions, including heart attack, stroke, cancer, depression, and Alzheimer's disease.

Getting More Omega-3s

To boost the omega-3 content of your diet and potentially reduce your risk of heart attack, cancer, and other conditions, you would be wise to fill your shopping cart with more omega-3—rich foods. In fact, unless you seek out foods high in omega-3 fats, you're apt to have a traditional American diet that's crowded with potentially damaging omega-6 fatty acids. Besides purslane, which isn't an option unless you plan to visit rural Greece in the near future or you have the "weed" in your garden, the following are some of the best and most readily available sources of omega-3 fats in the United States:

- *Fatty fish such as salmon, tuna, trout, herring, bluefish, sardines, and mackerel.* Eating healthy-fat "fatty" fish once or twice a week is an efficient way to get more omega-3s in your diet and reduce your risk of heart attack.

- *Walnuts.* Abundant in the Mediterranean diet, walnuts are a rich source of alpha-linolenic acid, a fat that converts to heart-

> **A Note from Dr. Jonas**
> FISHING FOR OMEGA-3S
>
> The American Heart Association recommends the consumption of fish as both an excellent source of omega-3 and a good protein source that's low in saturated fat.

healthy omega-3 fatty acids in the body. Add walnuts to salads, baked goods, appetizers, and sauces as they do in Greece, southern Italy, Spain, and France.

- *Canola oil.* Once purely a staple at health food stores, canola oil is now available at most supermarkets across the country (in case you're wondering, it comes from the seeds of a rape plant, which is in the mustard family). Reach for brands enriched with vitamin E (check the label), an antioxidant that's good for your heart and may also protect against prostate cancer. Since canola oil is bland tasting, it's also suitable for cooking and baking. For foods such as salad dressing that demand more flavor, consider doing a mix of canola oil and extra-virgin olive oil. But be sure to dole out both oils sparingly. Like olive oil, canola oil has 120 calories per tablespoon and can contribute to weight gain if consumed in excessive amounts.

- *Flaxseeds and flaxseed oil.* Both are available at health food stores and by mail order. Sprinkle ground flaxseed over salads, cereals, or into yogurt. Use flaxseed oil in homemade salad dressing.

Confused about which type of fat is healthy and which isn't? The table on page 20 can help you sort out the types of fat in your diet, what each does to your body, and the foods it's predominantly found in.

Fat Facts

FAT TYPE	KNOWN AS A	FOUND MOSTLY IN	EFFECT ON HDL/LDL CHOLESTEROL
Saturated fat	"Bad" fat	Whole-milk dairy products such as butter, cheese, milk, ice cream; red meat and poultry skin; vegetable oils such as coconut oil, cocoa butter, palm kernel oil and palm oil	Raises your body's cholesterol more than anything else in your diet.
Polyunsaturated fat	"So-so" fat	Corn oil, margarine	Lowers LDL (bad) cholesterol, but reduces HDL (good) cholesterol.
Mono-unsaturated fat	"Healthy" fat	Olive oil, canola oil	Typically lowers the unhealthy LDL cholesterol in your blood and raises healthy HDL cholesterol to reduce your risk of heart disease, when substituted for foods high in saturated fat.
Partially hydrogenated trans fatty acids	"Bad" fat	Stick margarine, shortening; processed pastries, cookies, and crackers; french fries and other deep-fried fast foods	Raises total cholesterol and LDL (bad) cholesterol. In very high amounts, may even lower HDL (good) cholesterol.
Omega-3 fatty acids	"Good" fat	Fatty fish such as salmon, tuna, trout, herring, bluefish, sardines, and mackerel; walnuts; canola oil; flaxseeds and flaxseed oil; leafy greens	Protects against heart disease and cancer; enhances brain functioning.
Omega-6 fatty acids	"So-so" fat	Corn, safflower, and sunflower oils	Heart healthy, but may block the health benefits of omega-3.

Mediterraneanize Your Meals

Throughout the Mediterranean, delicious, sun-soaked fruits and vegetables are a natural resource that have forever ruled the Mediterranean menu for simple reasons: Unlike meat, fruit and vegetables were inexpensive and readily available, often growing among the riches on a small farm, a sight still common in rural areas. Consequently, "what you'll see on the table if you go to somebody's grandmother's house in a rural village is 80 percent vegetables like zucchini, tomatoes, onions, eggplant straight from the garden," says Nikki Rose. Rose is a Greek American professional chef and director of the Washington, D.C.–based World Culinary Arts, an organization that educates American chefs on the food ways of Greece.

Throughout the Mediterranean in general, visitors frequently rave about the intensely flavored produce, bounty that's a product of the long growing season and a climate like California's central valley. In the south of France in the summer, for example, the apricot trees perfume the air. What do you look for after lunch in June? Apricots, of course. And the tomatoes. "They're blood red, so gloriously flavorful, you just drop dead when you taste one," says Lynn Kutner, a New York City cooking instructor who regularly summers in Provence. Mediterranean tomatoes even inspire rituals. In rural Greece, for example, dressing the fresh tomatoes with just the right proportion of olive oil to vinegar to seasoning is a dinner formality usually reserved for the eldest male member of a clannish household. "Not too much salt. More olive oil!" Nightly, the family members gathered around the table can't resist shouting out instructions on just how to properly adorn the prized fruit.

Food for Thought

In southern Italy in the 1960s, fruits and vegetables such as tomatoes, broccoli, and endive were the most commonly consumed foods, after bread and pasta. Today, Italians' love affair with produce continues. Visit Sicily, for example, and the locals are easy to spot. They're the ones examining the produce at the weekly farmers' market— picking it up, inhaling its aroma, and giving it a firm squeeze.

Healthy Peasant Food

Throughout the rural areas of the Mediterranean basin, you're still likely to be served meals of two-thirds steamed vegetables to one-third meat. In Greece, for example, the average consumption of produce remains at 400 grams a day (about four to five 3-ounce servings). In some areas of the Mediterranean, they even make a habit of drinking the nutrient-rich juice from which the vegetables have been steamed, which is considered, along with olive oil, a supreme tonic for vim and vigor.

As a rule, fresh-picked, deep-colored red, yellow, green, and purple produce offers the most nutrition value (and thus more potent disease-fighting power) per calorie. But you don't have to shop at a Mediterranean farmers' market to reap the health benefits of produce. In fact, it doesn't matter where you get your produce, whether it's fresh or frozen (canned is okay, too, although least preferred by registered dietitians), or even what color it is. Just get it in. After all, even lowly iceberg lettuce, previously much maligned for its lack of nutrient content, has something to offer: Studies have linked it to a lower risk of hip fractures in middle-aged and older women.

Top Produce Cancer Fighters from the Mediterranean

Apricots

Secret weapon: Impressive amounts of phytochemicals (plant chemicals) and the antioxidants vitamin C, lycopene, and beta-carotene, in addition to fiber. When fresh apricots aren't available, juice-packed canned apricots or dried apricots will do the job, although ounce per ounce, they tend to be higher in calories than their fresh counterpart.

Added bonus: Three medium fresh apricots have just 50 calories.

Broccoli, Brussels Sprouts, and Cauliflower

Secret weapon: Chemical substances that help rouse the cancer-fighting phase II detoxification enzymes in the body. Phase II detoxification enzymes are in *every* organ system in the body. They're your first line of defense against all the chemical carcinogens (cancer-causing agents) that come into your body. Common carcinogens include secondhand cigarette smoke, diesel fumes from trucks and buses, and PCBs, contaminants that may be in the water supply.

Added bonus: Broccoli contains cancer-protective phytochemicals called sulforaphane and indoles that seem to "mop up" toxins that promote cancer. *Tip:* If you're bored with broccoli, try its slightly bitter Italian cousin, broccoli raab, available in specialty markets and many supermarkets. Steam it just like you would regular broccoli, or sauté it with garlic in a little olive oil or canola oil.

Garlic and Onions

Secret weapon: Allyl sulfides, which trigger and improve your body's detoxification enzyme levels to inactivate carcinogens.

Added bonus: Allyl sulfides have been found to block enzymes in the stomach that cause chemicals to become active carcinogens in the body. You'll find garlic in numerous Mediterranean dishes—from the aioli and rouille sauces of southern France to the paella in Spain, hence the long braids of fresh garlic that adorn countless kitchens.

Oranges

Secret weapon: Folate and the antioxidant vitamin C. Just one orange provides an entire day's recommended dietary allowance for vitamin C.

Added bonus: Vitamin C helps your body absorb iron. Drinking orange juice, eating an orange, or consuming any vitamin-C–rich food with one that contains iron increases your body's iron absorption by at least 25 percent. Iron is especially important for women of child-bearing age. Iron helps carry oxygen to the blood and deliver it to cells. Without enough iron, you may feel sluggish and fatigued.

Tomatoes (especially cooked tomatoes as in tomato sauce and tomato paste)

Secret weapon: Cancer-fighting antioxidants such as beta-carotene, vitamin C, and the phytochemical lycopene (lycopene gives tomatoes their redness). In Italy, tomatoes are the second most prevalent source of vitamin C, after oranges. Lycopene is especially plentiful in processed tomato products such as canned tomatoes and tomato sauce, paste, juice, and soup.

Added bonus: Tomatoes and tomato products are a decent source of potassium, which is associated with a reduced risk of stroke.

GLOBAL EATING SECRET #4

Flavor Up Your Favorite Foods

From soups to sauces, salads, and vegetable and meat dishes, a traditional Mediterranean meal is a savory experience. In the southern Italian and southern French versions of the Mediterranean diet especially, herbs such as parsley, rosemary, thyme, basil, oregano, fennel, and

A Note from Dr. Jonas
HEALTHY EATING BEGINS IN THE STORE

Want to feed you and your family fast food, without succumbing to the nearest hamburger joint? To stick to a healthy diet (even though you swear there's no time), you need a strategy. *Tip:* When the going gets tough, don't get takeout. Run to the refrigerator or your cupboard.

With a well-stocked pantry, refrigerator, and freezer—filled with the kinds of foods mentioned throughout this book—you'll have the basis of countless healthy meals within arm's reach. You'll also be in and out of the supermarket in record time (but read food labels; you want to be sure of what you're buying). With a packed pantry, your grocery list will only need to include the healthy staples you're low on, plus the fresh foods you need each week, such as salad greens, fresh vegetables, milk, and eggs.

But to turn these ingredients into quick and healthy meals, you'll also need to set aside 20 minutes each week (the weekend is often a convenient time) to plan the menu for the week. There's no one right way to map out meals. Jot down ideas on scratch pieces of paper, or plot them out calendar style. Need ideas? See chapter 10 for recipes.

Food for Thought

Gobble up your garnish. In the United States, parsley adds what food professionals call "plate appeal." But in the Mediterranean, it's substance over style. Parsley is used in quantity to flavor salads and sauces. It also happens to be packed with important nutrients like vitamin C, folate, and cancer-fighting beta-carotene.

sage practically deserve their own food group. And rosemary, in particular, does a lot more than add a pleasantly piney flavor to meats, salads, and salad dressings.

Native to the region, rosemary grows wild in the Mediterranean and was once believed to cure various nervous system ailments. Now, researchers are discovering that there are constituents of rosemary that have very potent cancer-fighting antioxidant properties. Among other mechanisms, rosemary may increase the activity of detoxifying enzymes in the body that process foreign substances and carcinogens, especially those that lead to breast cancer. More research needs to be done, however, to determine exactly how much rosemary is necessary to reap these benefits.

In the meantime, experiment with rosemary when you're cooking. Add generous pinches of rosemary as well as other no-fat flavor enhancers such as thyme, basil, oregano, and vinegar (red, white, and zesty balsamic) to your recipes. Besides reducing your cancer risk, using herbs such as rosemary to season foods may curb your taste for salt and high-fat ingredients like butter.

——————— GLOBAL EATING SECRET #5 ———————

Eat More Beans

Long used as a meat substitute because they were relatively inexpensive, legumes such as fava beans, lentils, and chickpeas (garbanzos) are a staple in the traditional Mediterranean diet, which is perhaps another reason why chronic diseases like cancer and heart disease are less of a threat in this part of the world. Nutritionist Dorothea Klimis, Ph.D., a native of Greece, says that growing up, "we would have chicken or beef once a week. In the meantime, it would be fish and legumes—lentils, split peas and chickpeas."

Today in Greece, you'll also find lots of hummus, the chickpea dip, as well as white bean and garlic spreads for pita bread. The giant fava bean (a.k.a. broad bean) is also especially popular garnished with tomatoes, olive oil, and herbs. In the south of France, you'll find beans in the popular *pistou* soup, a rich vegetable bean mixture laden with a basil, garlic, and olive oil sauce. Lentils tossed in olive oil, garlic, and herbs are a frequent partner to meat. In southern Italy, white beans often make an appearance at meals in side dishes and quintessential soups like *pasta e fagioli* and minestrone.

To lower cancer risk, the American Institute on Cancer Research recommends eating more than seven servings a day of whole grains, legumes, roots, and tubers. But customarily, North Americans don't gravitate toward these kinds of foods. That may be one of the reasons why we average only 12 grams of fiber a day, less than half of the dietary recommendation. Beans and legumes are an efficient way to increase the fiber in your diet, which may help fight colon cancer. Just one cup of instant black bean soup, for example, provides 9 grams of fiber, about one-third of a day's fiber quota.

> ### A Note from Dr. Jonas
> ### STRIVE TO IMPROVE, NOT TO BE PERFECT
>
> Human beings can never be perfect, but we can always get better. Since a state of perfection is impossible for any of us to achieve, perfectionism is a destructive driving force for any behavior change. But knowing we can always get better can be motivating.
>
> If you deviate from the new healthy habits you're trying to establish, don't beat yourself up. To stay on the road to wellness, isolate your indiscretions. Say, "Okay, I just had a cheeseburger and french fries, and the chocolate cake. Now I'll go back to my regular routine." Keep in mind that it's normal to slip now and then. Overall, stability is what you're striving for—not the guilt-induced emotional roller coaster that perfectionism can bring on. If you find yourself giving up ("It's no use. I can't do this"), get support. For example, team up with a friend who'd also like to eat healthier, and go grocery shopping together. It's also a good idea to keep a food-and-exercise diary so you can track your progress and pinpoint problem areas.

There's more. The soluble fiber in beans also helps lower blood cholesterol and slows the breakdown of carbohydrates into glucose, which is important for people with Type 2 diabetes. Beans and legumes are also a significant and inexpensive source of protein, iron, and folate. Folate, a B vitamin, may protect against neural tube defects in newborns. It's also been shown to head off heart disease in adults by lowering blood levels of the amino acid homocysteine. Too much circulating homocysteine can irritate the lining of blood vessels, priming them for cholesterol and other fatty deposits. One cup of cooked lentils, for example, provides 360 micrograms (mcg) of folate (the entire day's requirement is 400 mcg).

Bean Opportunities

In case you're inspired, here are some simple solutions to up your bean intake, compliments of the people of the Mediterranean.

- Opt for the lentil or split pea soup over the cream of mushroom or chicken noodle varieties at the deli.

- When you're entertaining, serve black bean dip or hummus as appetizers (what the Greeks call *mezedakia*). Look for ready-made versions in your grocer's refrigerated specialty foods sections.

- Toss a can of black or white beans (well rinsed, to shed 30 to 40 percent of the sodium) into any soup or casserole.

- Add chickpeas (garbanzos) to your dinner salad. Don't forget to sprinkle a scoop of chickpeas on your salad any time you're at a salad bar.

- For a quick lunch, reach for instant black bean or lentil soup or vegetarian chili.

- For a change of pace, serve herbed bean salads or pureed beans as a side dish as an alternative to potatoes.

Besides beans, other excellent sources of fiber you should consider adding to your diet include bran cereal that has 5 grams of fiber or more per serving (check the label), and fresh fruits and vegetables such as pears and carrots.

Cooking with Beans and Lentils

Beans and lentils, legumes in general, are difficult to cook, right? Wrong. You can always open a can. Canned legumes offer as much fiber and nutrition as those that come dried. Canned beans and lentils can be high in sodium, but that can be easily remedied. Simply give them a good rinse before using to wash much of the sodium-based liquid away.

If you'd rather start from scratch, no problem. Simply rinse dried beans and soak in water (use four times as much water as beans).

A Note from Dr. Jonas
WORK IN A WORKOUT

Although the "low-risk coronary male" described in this chapter's introduction walked to work daily, walking and jogging aren't popular in Greece these days, and particularly not in cities like Athens, where buses are bursting at the seams with passengers and traffic clogs the streets daily. In Italy, on the other hand, approximately 35 percent of the population exercises at least once a week. This isn't enough to keep you fit, but it's a start. Favorite activities there include hiking, volleyball, jogging, and cycling.

(Lentils don't need soaking.) Throw away any beans that float, look moldy, or are otherwise discolored. *The leisurely method:* Soak beans overnight, pour off the soak water, then bring them to a slow boil in fresh water the next day. Reduce heat and simmer until beans are tender to taste. *The no-time-to-waste method:* Cover beans with cold water, bring to a boil and simmer for two minutes. Remove from heat, and let them stand for an hour. Then, bring them to a slow boil in fresh water, reduce heat, and simmer until tender.

GLOBAL EATING SECRET #6

Nuts Are Good for You

Nut trees flourish throughout the Mediterranean, and most residents with yards are apt to have an almond or walnut tree. Naturally, nuts are a popular Mediterranean snack and a key ingredient in many regional dishes and pastries such as baklava, phyllo pies, *dolmades* (grape leaves stuffed with rice, pine nuts, and currants), and *skordalia*, a savory walnut and garlic sauce. Greeks even have an official snack dish called *pastempo* (literally "to pass the time"), which is a plate of neatly composed piles of lightly roasted sunflower seeds, pumpkin seeds, and pistachios. And of course, what would pesto, the Italian basil-garlic sauce, be without pine nuts (pignoli)?

In the United States, nuts have gotten a bad rap because they're high in calories and unsaturated fat. But when it comes to fighting heart disease, the people of the Mediterranean, notorious for their nut consumption, may be on to something. According to results from the ongoing Nurses' Health Study published in the *British Medical Journal*, women who reported eating 5 ounces (or so) of nuts a week (about ½ cup) had a 35 percent reduction in heart disease risk compared with women who didn't eat nuts. The study credits the unsaturated fats found in nuts for improving the quality of blood fat levels, and states that nuts add other protective components to the diet, including protein, magnesium, vitamin E, fiber, and potassium. Other studies zeroing in on walnuts and almonds cite similar heart-healthy findings.

GLOBAL EATING SECRET #7

Pace Yourself with Alcohol

The people of the Mediterranean are known for their judicious alcohol consumption, which may help account for their lower rates of heart disease and longevity, thanks to the antioxidants and other healthful substances alcoholic beverages contain. Greece, Italy, Spain, and France are all significant wine-consuming countries. Wine derivatives such as *grappa*, a clear Italian spirit distilled from wine-grape skins, are also popular. Visit rural Greek regions like Patras and you're apt to be served a brandy-like homemade wine produced from the small vineyard on your host's property.

> **A Note from Dr. Jonas**
> PROTECT YOUR EYESIGHT
>
> The antioxidants found in wine as well as fruits and vegetables may protect you from macular degeneration, the leading cause of blindness in people over age sixty-five.

Throughout the Mediterranean, the tendency is to sip (not guzzle) alcoholic beverages, and to generally imbibe in moderation (drunkenness is rare). Drinking is also very seldom done without eating. In fact, order wine at a restaurant in Greece, and it's likely to arrive *with* your meal, not a minute before.

Downsizing Stress

The Mediterranean diet is more than diet. It's a lifestyle characterized by *la dolce vita* (the sweet life). Having a glass of wine over a convivial long-winded meal with family and friends is just one of the ways the people of the Mediterranean take time to relish life's meaningful moments. This laid-back, close-knit lifestyle may be just as relevant a factor behind the superior health statistics of the Mediterranean peoples as is their love of olive oil, fruits, vegetables, and legumes.

Studies show that psychological and social variables such as isolation, anxiety, and depression can not only influence your sense of well-being but also affect longevity. Unmanaged stress, in particular, can set off a hormonal chain of events that can have concrete effects on your long-term health.

Visit any country in the Mediterranean, and the souvenir you're apt to bring back with you is how healthy a less frenetic lifestyle feels. At first, however, if you're a typical multitasking American, the Mediterranean experience can be stress inducing. In the afternoon, shops will close for the midday siesta. The dinner "hour" can seem to last for days; the hospitality is that leisurely. "We have a saying in my family," says Nikki Rose, a Greek American professional chef. "Never go to a restaurant in Greece hungry." Friends who have toured Greece have commented on how, initially, they drum their fingernails to the quick and demand faster service. Then they give up and allow themselves to decompress, realizing that maybe the Mediterranean life-style isn't so bad, that in fact, maybe the people of this region know better.

All this downtime probably isn't practical for your everyday routine. But even a fraction of it can help extinguish the burnout that threatens our time-pressed lives. In fact, taking a breather throughout the day—even just a ten-minute walk here and there when stress mounts—can give your body and your mind a chance to rejuvenate. In the long run, to keep unmanaged stress from getting the best of you, studies show that the Mediterranean way—not being on "go" all the time—can be lifesaving.

Lesson Learned from the Mediterranean: Eat Right, but Don't Smoke

The traditional Mediterranean diet may be one of the healthiest in the world, but many people of the Mediterranean could be living on borrowed time. So far, their fiber- and antioxidant-rich diet may be protecting them from disease to some extent, but if it continues to change along its high-fat, North American track, they could be in danger. The reason: a high-fat diet and smoking are two major risk factors for heart disease, and many Mediterraneans are said to smoke like chimneys.

Indeed, smoking is rampant in Greece. Countless southern Italians and Spaniards are also heavy smokers. Likewise, smoking is so popular in France that restaurateurs are in the habit of creating impromptu no-smoking sections only at the request of customers by quickly hanging a sign above their table. Perhaps it's no coincidence then that the incidence of cancers of the lip, oral cavity, and pharynx (voice box) among French men is five times greater than among U.S. men.

Fortunately, smoking is currently on the decline among French men, es-pecially among higher-level executives, professionals, and academics. How-ever, it's rising among women. Those findings are similar to trends observed in Italy and Spain.

The Mediterranean Diet Pyramid

To help consumers decode the traditional Mediterranean diet and use it to improve their health, a team of nutrition professionals—the Oldways Preser-vation & Exchange Trust, the Harvard School of Public Health, and the

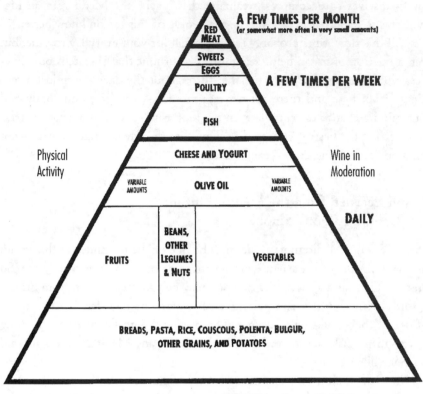

A FEW TIMES PER MONTH
(or somewhat more often in very small amounts)

A FEW TIMES PER WEEK

RED MEAT

SWEETS

EGGS

POULTRY

FISH

CHEESE AND YOGURT

Physical Activity

OLIVE OIL

VARIABLE AMOUNTS

VARIABLE AMOUNTS

Wine in Moderation

DAILY

FRUITS

BEANS, OTHER LEGUMES & NUTS

VEGETABLES

BREADS, PASTA, RICE, COUSCOUS, POLENTA, BULGUR, OTHER GRAINS, AND POTATOES

©1994 Oldways Preservation & Exchange Trust

The Traditional Healthy Mediterranean Diet Pyramid

Food for Thought

As the Mediterranean diet pyramid illustrates, yogurt (historically made from sheep's milk) is a prominent part of the traditional diet. Consider making it part of yours. A cup of U.S.-style plain low-fat or fat-free yogurt provides 35 to 40 percent of the recommended daily intake of calcium, which is a great way to get bone-building calcium to help prevent osteoporosis, a worldwide problem facing women and, to a lesser extent, men as they age.

World Health Organization Regional Office for Europe—developed the Mediterranean Diet Pyramid. This eating plan is similar to the Healthy American United States Department of Agriculture (USDA) Food Pyramid. It emphasizes a plant-based diet by placing grain-based foods as well as fruits and vegetables at its base. But here's how the two diets differ: With the traditional Mediterranean Diet Pyramid, red meat is at the tip of the pyramid, after sweets—in line with the custom in the Mediterranean in the 1950s and 1960s, when meat was scarce, it is on the menu just a few times a month. Also, olive oil is given a prominent central position on the pyramid—recommended to be consumed daily, which is why the traditional Mediterranean diet provides 35 to 40 percent of total daily calories from heart-healthy monounsaturated fat. Wine in moderation is also recommended. Daily exercise is also incorporated into the traditional Mediterranean pyramid, thanks to the physically hardworking people who in-spired it.

Incidentally, according to the World Health Organization, public health profession-als in Greece are working hard to promote and revitalize the traditional Mediterranean diet among the growing fast-food-and-butter-loving population. The Mediterranean diet pyramid was officially adopted in Greece as "the way to eat" in 1994.

The USDA Food Pyramid, on the other hand, recommends two to three daily servings of meat, poultry, fish, dry beans, eggs, and nuts. Fats, sweets, and alcoholic beverages are allowed, albeit "sparingly." Exercise is not ad-dressed in the USDA Food Pyramid, although it is discussed at great length in the Surgeon General's Report on Exercise and Health.

A Note from Dr. Jonas
GET MORE CALCIUM

To maximize your calcium absorption, be sure to eat plenty of calcium-rich foods that also contain vitamin D, such as fortified milk.

CHINA

Ancient Nutrition Secrets

Compared to the high-fat, sodium-laden convenience food that character-izes the North American diet, Chinese food *had* a healthy reputation. For years, Americans often equated Chinese food with "health food." But after Chinese food was put to the test by the folks at the Center for Science in the Public Interest, we're now more aware than ever that just because it's Chinese doesn't necessarily mean it's good for you. With crispy, tantalizing options such as General Tso's chicken, twice-cooked (read twice-fried) pork, and even deep-fried flounder—all weighing in at more than 75 grams of fat per serv-ing—ordering a Chinese meal in North America can mean consuming more fat then you'd need for an entire day, even more fat than in two Big Macs.

However, significant portions of the unhealthy foods found in Chinese restaurants in North America are not authentically Chinese. It was in the 1920s that Chinese restaurants first began to move beyond the boundaries of the Chinatowns that had sprung up in cities such as Los Angeles, San Fran-cisco, and New York. The restaurateurs who had emigrated from China dur-ing the latter part of the nineteenth century eventually realized that many Westerners would never go for their rice-based repertoire. So they invented what became the first standard Chinese restaurant menu, which had origins in Canton. Chow mein, chop suey, the pu pu platter, barbecued spare ribs, sweet-and-sour pork, egg rolls—even fortune cookies—are just a few of the menu items Chinese restaurateurs created to whet North American appetites. In the past twenty to thirty years, the "typical" Chinese restaurant menu has expanded considerably with the addition of other regional Chinese cuisines, such as those from Beijing, Shanghai, Szechuan, and Hunan.

Rice was the food of the country, to be respected in all its phases: the ripe grain in the husk, the paddy, glutinous rice, rice in the straw, hulled rice and cooked rice. To honor the farmers who planted, tilled, harvested and husked the rice, one was not supposed to leave even one kernel at the bottom of one's rice bowl.

—Pang-Mei Natasha Chang,
Bound Feet & Western Dress

Compared to traditional Chinese food, however, Americanized Chinese food continues to have its own distinct personality. Aside from what's served in Chinese tourist areas, "American Chinese restaurant cooking is much different from what we have in China," attests Lan Tan, a native of Taiwan, and owner of Lan Tan's Chinese Cooking School in Durham, North Carolina. She has spent nearly a decade teaching Americans who are trying to eat healthier how to cook "the Chinese way."

The difference? Tan contends that for one thing, U.S. Chinese restaurants use much more meat than do traditional Chinese. While *some* traditional Chinese dishes are fried, she admits, many are prepared with little more than a tablespoon or two of healthy-diet enemy number one—fat. "Cooking oil has always been an expensive commodity in China, so we don't do a lot of frying," Tan explains. Further, throughout China's history, political upheavals often disrupted agriculture and local trade networks. Fried foods and meat were customarily reserved for special occasions because the government often rationed cooking oil and meat. As a result, it wasn't uncommon for a Chinese family to stretch one pound of meat over an entire month's worth of eating. The majority of Chinese, especially in rural areas, thus had no choice but to direct their diet to the lower parts of the food chain and anoint rice, soybeans, and vegetables as their primary sustenance—foods that established the basis of their healthy diet.

Importing the Chinese Way

Today, the legacy of the authentic Chinese diet's inherent healthfulness triumphs. But to find proof, don't look to China's urban, modernized metropolises where certain Western eating trends have taken root. In Hong Kong, for example, the incidence rates of major chronic diseases such as heart disease, stroke, and cancer are climbing right along with burgeoning income levels and the rapid influx of Western-style restaurants.

Instead, venture deep into China's countryside, where an estimated 80 percent of the Chinese reside. In villages such as those found in rural Sichuan (Szechwan) province, where the rich fields of rice, wheat, corn, barley, potatoes, sugarcane, cotton, and tea are harvested, you'll see comparatively few obese Chinese, even though they generally consume roughly 300 more calories per day than do North Americans. There, the rates of many major, chronic diseases—including breast, colon, and rectal cancers—are fractions of the rates reported in the United States.

Unfortunately, deaths from cardiovascular disease in certain rural and urban parts of China are beginning to rival those of the United States. "But there are some regions in China in which breast cancer and heart disease are almost unknown," says T. Colin Campbell, Ph.D., professor of nutritional biochemistry at Cornell and director of the Cornell-China-Oxford Project on Nutrition, Health, and Environment, the most comprehensive project on diet and disease ever done. As part of an ongoing team study with the Chinese Institute of Nutrition and Health Hygiene, Campbell has been studying more than a hundred Chinese rural villages since the early 1980s. Death rates from breast cancer in China are four times lower than in the United States. Type 2 diabetes is also much less prevalent.

The health habits associated with these low chronic disease rates in China are based on traditions and economic conditions that span centuries. But you don't have to be a Chinese peasant, use chopsticks, or shop at an Asian market to reap this degree of good health. As this chapter will show you, with a few modifications, "the Chinese way" is available for importing. All it takes is an adventurous palate, some inventiveness in the kitchen, and the desire to stay healthy for the long haul.

A Note from Dr. Jonas
RACE AND BREAST CANCER

Breast cancer risk for a North American woman varies widely, depending on her racial and ethnic background. As the chart below shows, women living in the United States are more than four times as likely to die from the illness as are Chinese women who live in China and eat a traditional diet.

	Rate
American Women	21.1
Chinese Women	5.0

Lifetime age-adjusted rate per 100,000 women

- American Women
- Chinese Women

Source: *American Cancer Society, Surveillance Research, 1998; World Health Organization 1996.*

The Traditional Chinese Diet at a Glance

Low rates of many major chronic diseases

- Compared to North Americans, the Chinese report significantly lower rates of breast, colon and rectal, and lung cancers and a lower incidence of Type 2 diabetes.

Food for Thought

In 1980, the Chinese government enacted a one-child-per-family national policy to control population growth. Consequently, writes Yunxiang Yan in Golden Arches East, *"in most families, children are the object of attention and affection from up to half a dozen adults: their parents and their paternal and maternal grandparents. The demands of such children are always met by one or all of these relatives, earning them the title 'Little Emperor' or 'Empresses.' When a little Emperor says, 'I want to eat at McDonald's,' this means the entire family must go along."*

Although McDonald's can hardly be held responsible, childhood obesity is becoming a problem in China, especially in urban sprawls such as Hong Kong, where U.S.-style fast-food restaurants have proliferated.

Packed with produce; less meat, more grains

- The traditional Chinese diet revolves around produce. The Chinese typically parlay more than a pound of produce per capita into their daily routine.

- Low-fat complex carbohydrates such as rice take center stage in the Chinese diet, which may explain why the diet is comparatively lower in fat. However, as the Chinese develop a taste for meat and Western-style restaurants become more common in China, the amount of fat the Chinese consume is increasing along with their risk of cardiovascular and other diseases.

Tea is the beverage of choice

- Tea, rich in disease-fighting antioxidants, is the traditional beverage of choice in China and has been for centuries.

Too high in sodium

- Sodium, principally from soy sauce and MSG (monosodium glutamate), is an element of the traditional Chinese diet that North Americans shouldn't try to emulate. High sodium intakes have been associated with comparatively high hypertension incidence rates in China.

GLOBAL EATING SECRET #8

Give Your Diet the Power of Produce

If you're like most North Americans, vegetables don't top your list of favorite foods. According to the National Cancer Institute, the average American adult consumes 4.5 servings of fruits and vegetables a day, which beats our record of only 3.9 daily servings in the late 1980s. Five to nine servings per day of these combined food groups are recommended for a healthy diet. Yet, the produce we consume isn't always in the healthiest form. According to USDA food consumption surveys, the potato is the most popular vegetable in America, and 50 percent of the time it's in the form of french fries.

On the other hand, the Chinese diet features, among others, deep-colored cruciferous (the cabbage family) greens such as Chinese cabbage, bok choy, mustard greens, and broccoli, which are packed with the disease-fighting antioxidant vitamins C and E as well as lutein, a cancer-fighting carotenoid that gives these richly colored vegetables their pigment. Epidemiological studies have found that cruciferous vegetables also contain organic compounds that may increase the activity of enzymes involved in detoxifying some carcinogens (cancer-causing agents). They may also affect estrogen metabolism and protect against estrogen-related cancers such as those of the breast and the uterus.

"The traditional Chinese diet is essentially one that consists chiefly of plant foods and only small amounts of fish, poultry and only occasionally red meat," says Dr. Campbell.

The Health Benefits of Antioxidants

To reduce your risk of cancer, studies show that antioxidants can help your body fight the chemical reactions that can lead to this dreaded killer. Ironically, one of the biggest dangers to the body is a molecular form of oxygen that's the very element we need for survival. In the oxygen we breathe, which is used to support life, each atom contains a pair of electrons. As we metabolize food and the body goes through its normal processes, however, some oxygen molecules shed one electron. They thus become "rogue" molecules called *free radicals.* Free radicals can attack healthy cells of all kinds, hoping to steal an electron from an atom in the cell to stabilize themselves. If not neutralized by antioxidants, which may donate an electron to free radicals without involving cells, free radicals are thought to damage cell DNA, laying the groundwork for cancer and potentially a host of other equally formidable diseases.

Fruits and vegetables, however, have a lot more going for them—and for you—besides antioxidants. As you're probably aware, they contain fiber, which may reduce your risk of colon cancer if you eat enough of it. The general recommendation: Aim for a diet that provides 20 to 30 or more grams of fiber a day. Phytochemicals such as indoles and sulforaphane are also provided by fruits and vegetables. These compounds are neither vitamins nor minerals, but studies show they may reduce the risk of breast cancer by activating the anticancer enzymes in the body.

Maybe you never outgrew the dislike of vegetables you may have had as a child. Or maybe your diet is centered on convenience foods. To reap the

Food for Thought

A common Chinese cure-all for the flu or a cold is a watery rice elixir called congee *—a diluted porridge of boiled rice and water. Congee is also a popular breakfast food in China as well as in Japan and Thailand.*

Chinese diet's health benefits, Dr. Campbell urges you to "make your food choices as varied as possible. The closer you get to a plant-based diet, the better off you'll be."

We all know that eating our vegetables is good for us. But maybe we just can't do it within the confines of a Western-style diet. That's where Chinese cooking can be a big help to you in becoming a healthier global eater. Here are several important steps you can take to give your diet the produce power the Chinese have been wielding for ages.

- **Develop a game plan.** To make sure fruits and vegetables make it into your shopping cart, plan menus that include fruits and vegetables. To make life interesting, experiment with exotic options such as bok choy, Swiss chard, papayas, mangoes, raspberries, blueberries, fresh pineapple, artichokes, sweet potatoes, celery root, broccoli raab, and turnips. For best flavor, variety, and quality, buy in season—a factor that's generally determined by price. Seasonal items are often the best deal in the market.

- **Start your day with a double.** As a rule, the earlier in the day you start chipping away at your quota of five to nine servings of fruits and vegetables as recommended by the National Cancer Institute, the easier it will be to get those servings in. Begin your day with 12 ounces of juice such as orange, grapefruit, or tomato, which is double the usual serving size, and you'll get two servings before you even leave the house. In general, a serving size equals ½ cup of a cooked fruit or vegetable, 1 cup of something raw, one medium-size piece of whole fruit, or ¾ cup of juice.

- **Stash produce in your desk drawer.** That way, you'll be ready when hunger strikes at work. With fruits and vegetables on deck, the vending machine will lose its luster. It's easy to pack raisins, cans of fruit or vegetable juice, and whole pieces of sturdy fruit such as apples, bananas, or pears.

- **Sneak produce into meals.** Add fruits and vegetables to the foods you already eat. For example, top off your morning cereal or yogurt with bananas, berries, or peaches. Layer sandwiches with dark leafy greens such as spinach and watercress; order your burger or chicken or fish sandwich with extra lettuce, tomato, and onion. Roll bean sprouts, shredded cabbage, and slices of green or red pepper into tortillas or flat bread; heap salsa onto low-fat tortilla chips; toss peas, tomatoes, onion, celery, carrots, and peppers into a salad. Pitch mushrooms, peppers, zucchini, onions, and carrots into pasta sauce, meat loaf, soup, stew, and chili.

- **Reorganize your refrigerator.** What we eat is often what we see first when we look in places where we store food. With this in mind, move sealed bags of baby carrots, precut red and green pepper strips, and broccoli florets to the top shelf instead of hiding them in the crisper bin. Slide a container of hummus, *baba ghanoush* (pureed eggplant, tahini, olive oil, lemon juice, and garlic), or nonfat salad dressing next to the vegetables (hint, hint). You'll be enticed as soon as you open the refrigerator door.

- **Choose fruit for dessert.** Cloying concoctions such as brownie chocolate cheesecake and pecan pie after a meal are a bit of a head scratcher to the Chinese; their culture doesn't participate in the postmeal ritual we call dessert. Fresh fruit, on the other hand, is the unofficial national treat of China. Of course, because it has no fat and fewer calories than most classic Western desserts, fruit is a much better nutritional deal. The fiber it contains may even help you digest your meal. If you find fresh fruit too puritanical for your tastes, try fresh fruit sorbet. With less fat than frozen yogurt and only 100 calories per half cup, brands made with fruit juice (check the label) are a sweet way to get vitamin C. (By the way, tastes do change. If you opt for fresh fruit for dessert once a week or so, you may find yourself seeking it out more often.)

  If you're dying for something more traditionally sweet but still healthy, seek out fruit and vegetable delights such as reduced-fat carrot cake, chocolate

---

A Note from Dr. Jonas
GETTING GOOD AT GOAL SETTING

To become a lifelong healthy eater, you need to be clear about what you want to accomplish and why. In other words, you need to set the right goal or goals for yourself. In terms of eating, those goals may focus on the content of your diet, your weight (either too much or too little), or both. To set realistic goals, think about why you want to make changes and what you expect to accomplish. For example, do you want to look better, feel better, and feel better about yourself? Or are you interested in reducing your future risk of one or more diseases? Or do you want to lose weight?

Another important part of goal setting is to understand for whom you want to accomplish your goals. Is it to please someone else, or to please yourself? If the goals you set are yours, you significantly increase the likelihood that your efforts will lead to a lifelong pattern of healthy eating.

zucchini cake, blueberry or apple pie, or pumpkin cheese cake (low fat, of course) at farm stands and bakeries.

―――――――― GLOBAL EATING SECRET #9 ――――――――
Think Complex Carbs First

For years now, we've been hearing in the news and in the media how important it is for our health to eat more grains such as rice, whole-grain breads, and cereals such as oatmeal. Technically speaking, these foods are complex carbohydrates made from chains of simple sugars that provide vitamins and minerals as well as energy. They also tend to be low in fat and high in fiber, which can aid digestion and reduce your risk of developing heart disease and colon cancer. As you may know, heart disease is the number-one killer of both men and women in North America. Colon cancer is also deadly; it kills over 45,000 people every year in the United States. Studies estimate that men and women who eat the traditional Western diet, which features red and processed meats and refined grains and sugars, and is low in fresh fruits and vegetables, double their overall colon cancer risk.

According to food consumption surveys, most of us still don't get it. We should be consuming 60 percent of our calories from complex carbohydrates. While roughly 39 percent of our calories come from grain products, an equal number come from refined carbohydrates such as sugars and sweeteners, which have zero disease-fighting power.

Rice Predominates

Enter the Chinese, who have been relying on rice and wheat products as the core of their diet since early antiquity. Average annual rice consumption in China totals a whopping 200 to 400 pounds per capita—about 800 percent more rice per year than is consumed in the United States. Their secret? They make grains such as rice the entrée and use meat as merely a way to flavor it.

This dietary role reversal has been part of their culinary tradition, called *cai-fan,* for centuries. "Food in China is mainly divided into two parts," explains Yanrong Liu, a food and nutrition graduate student at the University of Arkansas, who hails from the Shandong province in northeastern China, near the Yellow Sea. "One part is *fan* (literally cooked rice), which includes rice, steamed breads, sweet potatoes and rolls. *Cai* is the other part, a mix of vegetables and a little bit of meat. *Fan* is usually served in individual bowls and *cai* is served on the table for the whole family. This is the tradition."

In northern China, dumplings and breads frequently stand in for rice. But in southern China, the rice habit is so "ingrained," its mealtime absence is keenly felt, even for modernized Chinese. "We now live in America, and have plenty of high-quality meats available. But if we don't eat *fan* during a meal, we feel like we didn't eat at all," says Liu, who, along with her husband, owns a Chinese restaurant in Fayetteville, Arkansas. Lan Tan has similar sentiments: "My husband and I eat rice nearly every meal. Personally, if I don't eat rice every day, I don't feel good."

While any complex carbohydrate will do the job of displacing meat and other high-fat, calorie-dense foods, rice has become the principal means of sustenance for over half the world's population because it's such a nutritious and wholesome grain. One-half cup of white rice, for example, contains only 82 calories (89 for brown rice). Cholesterol free with only a trace of fat, rice is also low in sodium, gluten-free, nonallergenic, and easy to digest. It's one of the best sources of complex carbohydrates. The Chinese tradition of relying on grains such as rice as the main course is one of the chief health habits to consider importing into your diet. Of course, if you'd rather stick to more familiar territory, any grain-based food will do—pasta, couscous, oatmeal, and whole-grain bread, for example.

And here's another trick the Chinese use: When you think about what you're going to eat, first ask, "What grain shall I have?" Aim for a ratio of two-thirds complex carbohydrates to one-third meat, if any. To safeguard your intentions, buy meat in quarter- to half-pound packages; ask the butcher to divvy up a larger package for you.

Food for Thought

In traditional Chinese cooking, meat and vegetables have equal footing; both are considered main dishes. Three or more main vegetable dishes may be served at one meal, especially at dinner.

A Note from Dr. Jonas

CHOPSTICKS—THE ULTIMATE DELAY TACTIC

It takes roughly twenty minutes for the sensation of fullness to register in your brain. To downshift your eating by at least 25 percent so you'll be less inclined to go back for seconds, save the chopsticks from your Chinese takeout and use them at home regularly.

The Varieties of Rice

While many varieties of rice and rice products are available in supermarkets across North America—everything from flavored rice mixes to specialty rices such as Texmati or basmati—you will most commonly find one of two basic types: white or brown. White rice has been completely milled so that the outer husk, the bran, and most of the germ have been removed. To compensate for the nutrients lost during milling, white rice grown in the United States is enriched with iron and the B-vitamins thiamin and niacin. Brown rice, on the other hand, has the outer hull removed but still retains the nutrient-rich bran layers that give it tan coloring and a nutlike flavor.

Although both types are good sources of complex carbohydrates, protein, thiamin, niacin, and iron, brown rice is the marginal nutritional winner. Not only does it pack more cholesterol-lowering fiber than regular white rice does, but it's also the only form of rice containing the antioxidant vitamin E. Healthy doses of vitamin E may protect against heart disease by preventing LDL, the "bad" cholesterol, from oxidizing and causing artery damage.

In addition to white and brown rice, which comes in long, medium, or short grains, many instant mixes and exotic grains are available in most supermarkets. Here are some of the most popular ones:

Basmati. An aromatic rice popular in India and in Middle Eastern countries, this rice swells into long, thin grains when cooked. Types of U.S.-grown rice that are similar to basmati include Texmati, Wehani, and Wild Pecan. You can substitute basmati for regular rice in any recipe.

Jasmine. In Thailand, nearly every meal contains jasmine rice; all other dishes are considered an accompaniment. With a soft, moist texture, jasmine clings together when cooked.

Flavored rice mixes. These packaged grains typically come with seasonings or sauces. Many contain processed brown or white rice that cooks quickly. Although generally nutritious, beware of mixes with high sodium content. Check the label—some may have 1,000 milligrams per a ¾-cup serving, which is about half the recommended maximum daily intake. To reduce sodium, try using only half the contents of the seasoning packet when cooking.

Cooking with Rice

Contrary to popular belief, rice is a cinch to prepare. Here's how: Just double the amount of water, chicken broth, or vegetable juice in a recipe to the amount of uncooked rice—say, 2 cups of water to 1 cup of rice. Cover and bring to a boil, then simmer until fluffy, about 20 minutes (45 minutes for brown rice). One cup of uncooked rice yields about 3 cups cooked, and costs an average of just seven cents per ½ cup serving. For extra flavor, add herbs and spices such as ginger, chili powder, garlic, basil, or thyme. For more fiber and nutrients, toss in a bevy of diced vegetables.

GLOBAL EATING SECRET #10

Demote Meat at Mealtime

Using meat as merely a flavoring agent is a Chinese tradition that dates back to the T'ang dynasty (A.D. 618–906). Known as China's Golden Age, it was then, note historians, that Chinese cuisine began to evolve into an association between food and medicine. Chinese herbal pharmacologists determined what could and could not be eaten, when, how, in what quantities, and in which combinations. Meat, particularly the flesh of domestic animals such as cattle, pigs, and sheep, was unanimously deemed damaging to health.

In some regions of China today, that disdain for meat still prevails. "Many Chinese think consuming a large quantity of meat at one time is bad for your health," says Yanrong Liu, the Chinese restaurateur in Arkansas. A typical entrée in China's rural villages is meat hidden among a mound of vegetables. "Even I forget just how healthy Chinese food really is until my mother visits from Taiwan," adds Lan Tan, who admits to becoming a bit more Westernized since coming to the United States more than a decade ago. "My mother will use one-third pound of meat to feed six people."

Economic circumstances, more than any other factor, may underlie China's use of meat as a condiment. A study by Barry M. Popkin of the University of North Carolina School of Public Health that involved 16,000 Chinese from various economic levels, concluded that as income rises, the Chinese are apt to eat less rice and wheat products and more fresh fruit, dairy products, high- and low-fat red meat, poultry, eggs, fish, and seafood. In China's urbanized, Westernized sprawls such as Hong Kong, in which meat is a once-a-day affair, the rates of hypertension and stroke are growing.

"In Hong Kong, people are going crazy about meat," confirms Georgia Guldan, Ph.D., associate professor of nutrition at the Chinese University in Hong Kong. "At lunch time, you'll find office workers ordering entrées such as 'Barbecued Plate,' a small bed of rice topped with several pork chops, a slice of ham, and another piece of meat," she says. You'll also spot schoolchildren munching on Big Macs. "Meat is such a highly prized food because formerly only the very affluent could afford to eat it," she says.

A Note from Dr. Jonas
MEAT IS OVERRATED

Meat, especially red meat such as beef and pork (although poultry isn't entirely innocent), tends to be high in fat, especially artery-clogging saturated fat, which elevates blood cholesterol and increases your risk of cardiovascular disease. Fat may also contribute to your risk of cancer; at 9 calories per gram (compared with only 4 calories per gram of protein or carbohydrate), fat is a dense nutrient that appears to be linked to rapid cellular growth, although no conclusive studies have yet cemented the fat-cancer relationship.

In jumbo proportions, the protein found in meat may also be a health hazard. In one study, adults with high cholesterol who replaced half their meat consumption with vegetables (which also contain protein, but in vegetable form) dropped their cholesterol levels 6 percent. And because protein can cause calcium to be excreted, a high-protein diet has also been tied to an increased risk of the bone-thinning disease osteoporosis.

In China's rural villages, however, where meat is still considered a luxury and the traditional rice-based cuisine is standard fare, the rates of major chronic diseases remain decidedly low. To counteract this Western influence in China's cities, where many of China's trends emerge and take hold, the Chinese government has initiated damage control by launching a public health campaign to weave nutrition into the public consciousness. North America, and its high rates of major chronic diseases, are fueling their resolve as if to say, "If you're not careful, this is where you're headed."

Meat Isn't All Bad

Despite the decree by Chinese pharmacologists, red meat, chicken, and turkey aren't demons in your diet—if consumed in reasonable amounts. In fact, most meat is rich in iron, zinc, magnesium, several B vitamins (with the exception of folate, the food form of folic acid), phosphorus, and protein. But if and when you do eat meat, eating the Chinese way dictates that you consume meat in near appetizer quantities—no more than two 3-ounce servings of meat a day. (One standard serving of meat is about the size of your debit card.) Here's how to make the most of streamlined meat meals using the Chinese approach:

- **Give vegetables and grains entrée status.** Crowd your plate with vegetables and grains such as rice or pasta. Consider meat the flavoring rather than the main attraction. Along with the meat, have a baked potato *and* spinach, for example, or a tossed salad *and* asparagus. Once a week, it's a good idea to go all out and prepare a totally vegetarian meal such as vegetable lasagna or baked white or sweet potatoes with vegetarian toppings.

- **When you do eat meat, choose low-fat cuts and amp up their flavor.** Marinate them for at least 15 minutes before cooking. The acid in a marinade (many marinade recipes call for lemon or lime juice, wine or vinegar) can tenderize low-fat cuts. Good choices usually include cuts with "loin" or "round" in their name, as in round steak or pork loin, as well as white meat without the skin.

- **Trim all visible fat from meat before cooking.** You'll save an average of 11 grams of fat (roughly 100 calories) per serving when you pre-trim the fat. Any remaining fat will migrate into the meat during cooking.

- **Skip the skin.** Unlike cows, pigs, and sheep, who store most of their fat in and around the muscles we eat as meat, chickens, turkeys, and ducks store their fat just under their skin. Therefore, remove the skin from chicken and turkey before cooking and you'll save an additional 100 calories per 3-ounce serving. When roasting whole birds, leave on the skin if you wish so the meat doesn't dry out; just throw away the skin before eating the bird.

- **Don't fill up on chicken.** It's not innocent. Although chicken tends to be lower in fat than beef or pork, studies show that the saturated fat contained in chicken, especially in the dark meat, can still raise your blood cholesterol, and ultimately increase your risk of heart disease.

- **Order ethnic.** Go ahead, order Chinese. But skip the deep-fried Chinese American fare such as General Tso's chicken. Instead, head for the vegetarian section of the menu and eat the way the traditional Chinese do. Look for entrées made with napa cabbage, bok choy, spinach, and broccoli, which are packed with vitamins A and C as well as fiber and phytochemicals. If meat is a must, order your chicken or beef mixed with vegetables such as snow peas, green and red peppers, string beans, or zucchini. And don't forget to showcase your plate with an extra bowl of white or brown rice.

Asian Diet Pyramid

As an alternative to the USDA Food Pyramid, the Asian Diet Pyramid might suit your needs and your palate. Created by Cornell and Harvard University researchers in collaboration with the nonprofit organization Oldways Preservation & Exchange Trust, the Asian Diet Pyramid reflects the traditional, plant-based rural diets of Asia. As mentioned earlier, the Asian diet may be linked to the low rates of certain cancers, heart disease, obesity, and

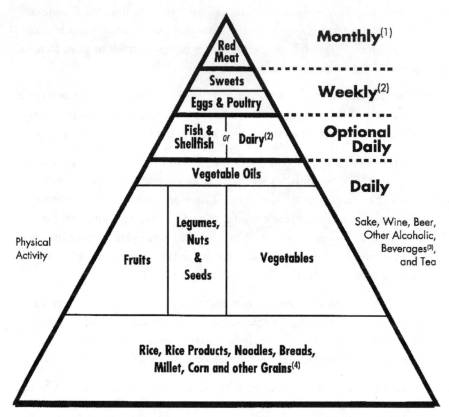

The Healthy Asian Diet

The following notes appear within the diagram:

Monthly[1]

Weekly[2]

Optional Daily

Daily

Red Meat

Sweets

Eggs & Poultry

Fish & Shellfish or Dairy[2]

Vegetable Oils

Fruits

Legumes, Nuts & Seeds

Vegetables

Rice, Rice Products, Noodles, Breads, Millet, Corn and other Grains[4]

Physical Activity

Sake, Wine, Beer, Other Alcoholic, Beverages[3], and Tea

©1995 Oldways Preservation & Exchange Trust

(1) Or more often in very small amounts.
(2) Dairy foods are generally not part of the healthy, traditional diets of Asia, with the notable exception of India. In light of current nutrition research, if dairy foods are consumed on a daily basis, they should be used in low to moderate amounts, and preferably low in fat.
(3) Wine, beer and other alcoholic beverages should be consumed in moderation and primarily with meals, and avoided whenever consumption would put an individual or others at risk.
(4) Minimally refined whenever possible.

osteoporosis in Japan and China. Clearly, carbohydrates dominate this diet while meat and sweets take a backseat. (By the way, the Japanese are known for indulging in Western-style sweets such as strawberry shortcake or pastries about four o'clock each workday afternoon to break the long fast until dinner—not exactly a habit you'll want to emulate.) A small amount of vegetable oil and a moderate amount of plant-based beverages including green or black tea, sake, beer, and wine are allowed. Daily physical exercise is also stressed (yes, in the Asian approach to healthy eating, physical activity is considered an integral part of the equation). Nearly absent are dairy products, because traditionally, the Asian diet has been dairy-free. Even so, Asian countries report lower rates of osteoporosis than do North American countries. Until more is known about the nature of osteoporosis and its relation to diet, however, North American women are strongly advised to get plenty of calcium in their diet.

GLOBAL EATING SECRET #11

Try Wok-Style Cooking with a Skillet or Dutch Oven

The wok is one of the most universally recognized utensils in the Chinese kitchen, and one of the best ways to stir-fry, often translated as "fast-fry," a cooking method that quickly sears meat and vegetables with the option of using very little added fat. But you don't need a traditional Chinese wok to stir-fry at home. In fact, because of the wok's concave design, it is argued that the wok makes little sense for flat Western stove tops. (In China, woks traditionally sat in cylindrical fire pits, with heat from all sides cooking the food.) It makes more sense for North American cooks to use a Dutch oven or large skillet with a tight-fitting lid so steam can't escape. (Do not use a Teflon-lined pot.) Here is a step-by-step guide to low-fat wok cooking the North American way.

1 Dice a slew of your favorite vegetables, such as onions, mushrooms, red and green peppers, carrots, scallions, cauliflower, broccoli, spinach, and bok choy, into small quarter-size pieces. Set aside. (In traditional China, small pieces were a must for wok cooking to save on cooking time and, thus, cooking fuel.)

2 Chop flavor makers such as garlic, ginger, scallions, and hot peppers. Set aside.

3 Cut tofu, seafood, chicken breast, pork or beef into ¼-inch pieces. Aim for double the amount of vegetables to meat, poultry, tofu, or fish. Set aside.

4 Heat a seasoned pan until you see a light smoke come off the sides. Your pan needs to be very hot since the point is to sear the food surfaces and seal the juices in. Add 1 tablespoon of oil or chicken broth to the pan. Swirl the pot to glaze it with the oil. If you're using a traditional wok,

toss in a bit of whatever is to go into the pot first. When the item sizzles, it's about 350°F and it's ready.

5 Add flavor makers: garlic, ginger, scallions, and/or hot peppers. Cook for 10 seconds, mashing with the back of a spatula to draw out flavor.

6 Add the meat, seafood, or tofu, and cook until about three-quarters done. Remove from pan; cover and keep warm.

7 Add 1 tablespoon of oil to the pan; heat it for about 1 minute or until hot. Add longer-cooking vegetables such as carrots, cauliflower, onions, and peppers, and cook until tender crisp.

8 Leaving the first batch of vegetables in the pan, add faster-cooking vegetables such as asparagus, green beans, broccoli, cabbage, mushrooms, and summer squash. Cook until tender crisp.

9 Add reserved cooked meat, seafood, or tofu. Stir-fry about 1 minute more.

10 Serve on a king-size bed of white or brown rice.

GLOBAL EATING SECRET #12

Develop a Taste for Tea

A Note from Dr. Jonas
THE MAGIC OF MOTIVATION

Everyone talks about motivation. You know, "How do I get motivated?" "One day, I'm motivated, the next day, I'm not. How do I keep it up?" "Once I get motivated, watch out. Things are going to change around here." But just what is motivation, anyway? Many of us talk about motivation as if it were a tangible thing, something you can go to a mall and buy—if only there were a store that sold it. But, in fact, motivation is a process that links a thought or feeling to the taking of an action.

Travel to China and you'll see North American advertising for coffee. Television and newspaper ads as well as billboards have given coffee status-symbol prestige. As alluring as coffee is in China, however, "The Chinese really don't have a taste for it," says Georgia Guldan, the Hong Kong nutrition professor. The Chinese version of coffee is and has traditionally been tea. "At any business meeting, you can always count on tea and an orange," attests Stephanie Holaday, professor of nursing at Catholic University in Washington, D.C., who spent months in Beijing and Shanghai studying Chinese family public policy.

Tea originated in China some four thousand years ago, and it's "steeped" in Chinese tradition. Grown principally in Taiwan, tea's original purpose was to mask the flat taste of the water the Chinese boiled to prevent illness from contamination. "But now the reason many Chinese people drink tea is because it's a healthy beverage," says Verna Tang, of the Chinese Information and Culture Center in New York City. Tang, a native of Taiwan, believes that tea helps prevent cancer. Some Chinese believe that a postmeal cup of tea helps cleanse the body.

Whether the majority of Chinese drink tea for its purported health properties is debatable. But Tang may be on to something. Research suggests that tea may be a powerful cancer fighter because it contains polyphenol antioxidants, a class of nutrients that is thought to protect the body against free-radical cell damage.

"Tea modifies enzymes in the liver to alter our biochemical defense mechanisms to produce a protective effect against cancer. It may also help halt heart disease by deoxidizing and disarming LDL cholesterol, the 'bad' artery-clogging cholesterol," says John H. Weisburger, Ph.D., of the American Health Foundation, a medical research organization in New York City.

Scientifically speaking, motivation is a state of mind such as an emotion, a desire, an idea, or an intellectual understanding, or a psychological, physiological, or health need mediated by a mental process, that leads to the taking of one or more actions.

It's important to understand that motivation is something that goes on internally, rather than something you can get from somewhere or somebody else. It's also important to understand that in most of us, in terms of our own health, the process we call motivation is always there. The problem for many of us, however, is that it's not always activated. It's sometimes blocked or inhibited by denial or previous failures. You know you're at this point when you make excuses such as "I have a slow metabolism," or "I come from a family of junk food addicts." Deep down, however, subtle warning signs are probably going off that you need to do something: Your clothes are tight; your doctor tells you that your cholesterol or blood pressure is high; you're worried that your diet is eventually going to take its toll.

In many instances, getting motivated means nothing more than breaking through internal barriers. To overcome your motivation minimizers, don't turn a deaf ear to those signals. Write a pro/con list about why you want to change your diet, and learn as much as you can about the benefits of a healthy diet.

It's Time for Tea

Black teas such as Earl Grey, English Breakfast, and regular Lipton, which are commonly drunk in North America, come from leaves that are fermented, then heated and dried to yield a dark red-brown brew. Green tea, favored among the Chinese and the Japanese, is produced from tea leaves that are steamed and dried but not fermented. They yield a beverage of a green-yellow hue and a flavor closer to that of the actual leaf. Both green and black tea offer protective effects, Weisburger says. (Sorry, herb tea enthusiasts. You won't reap these rewards from that beverage because it isn't made from tea leaves at all, but from an infusion of various herbs, flowers, and spices.)

How does tea work its wonders? "Because tea comes from a plant, it's in essence a vegetable extract," says Dr. Weisburger. Drinking tea is akin, for example, to drinking broccoli juice instead of eating the stalks.

How much tea to drink to reap health benefits is subjective, but Weisburger suggests 3 to 5 cups of black or green tea a day, an amount he says is equivalent to two servings of vegetables. If the caffeine content in tea is a worry (a 6-ounce cup of tea contains about 35 milligrams of caffeine, one-third the amount in a 6-ounce cup of coffee), switch to decaffeinated tea, which is usually available where tea is sold.

Taking the Opportunity to *"Yum Cha"*

Tea drinking sparks rituals among the Chinese and many other cultures. From about 6:30 A.M. to 2:00 P.M. daily, if time allows, the Chinese (especially those from Canton) are known to *yum cha,* to have tea at a Chinese teahouse. Visit a Chinatown in the United States and you, too, can partake in this Cantonese tradition. At teahouses in New York City's Chinatown, such as Nom Wah Tea Parlor on Doyers Street or Hao Shih Chieh on Catherine Street, you can expect to be served herb teas like jasmine and *sow mei* (chrysanthemum flower tea), or the basic *boolay,* otherwise known as black tea.

If you wish to be traditional, drink these teas hot, sans sugar or milk. When you're ready for more, give the teapot lid a flip up to signal to the waiter that your teapot is dry. To act like an insider, try these hand signals: If you'd like more jasmine tea, rub your finger under your nose as if you're drawing an imaginary mustache, and your waiter will fill your pot. For more *sow mei,* brush your brow from left to right with your right index finger. Want more chrysanthemum tea? Cup your fingers upright into flower petals. For more black tea, give your right earlobe a tug.

Besides being served tea at the Chinese teahouse, you can expect to be served dim sum (literally, "little tastings"), a series of savory bite-size snacks. From a rolling cart that a waiter brings every so often to your table, expect to be offered *Ja Fun Chow,* dumplings with minced pork and peanuts; *Char Shiu Bao,* small buns filled with roast pork; *Wu Gok,* mashed taro root filled with diced pork then rolled in starch and fried; and *Cheung Gwin,* spring rolls.

Don't know what to try or even what's being offered? Just point to what looks good and the waiter will take your cues. But take heed. The Chinese are accustomed to using all parts of an animal in cooking. And *Foon Jow*, a dim sum delicacy that looks like ruddy brown lumps, may not be to your liking. It's chicken feet. Feeling adventurous? Go ahead and give it a try. But keep in mind that *Foon Jow* is designed to be savored for a minute or two then promptly deposited into your napkin.

The Chinese teahouse is a place to enjoy much-needed downtime with friends and fellow workers and to take refuge from the demands of the outside world. For recommended teahouses in the United States, call the Chinese Cultural Association in cities that have a Chinatown, such as New York, Boston, Los Angeles, or San Francisco.

GLOBAL EATING SECRET #13

Don't Use Too Much Salt or Soy Sauce

Soy sauce is an extremely important ingredient in Chinese cooking used to flavor soups, sauces, marinades, meat, fish, and vegetables. It's also one of the few rather *un*healthy components of the cuisine. Made by fermenting boiled soybeans and roasted wheat or barley, this salty sauce has a dark side: Both soy sauce and MSG (monosodium glutamate), a common Chinese flavor enhancer derived from seaweed, vegetables, or sugar beets, have been implicated in boosting the rates of heart disease in China and Japan. MSG contains only one-third the amount of sodium as salt and imparts a distinctive savory, meaty flavor. One tablespoon of soy sauce, on the other hand, has 830 milligrams of sodium. But your body only needs about ¼ teaspoon of sodium (535 milligrams) a day to function properly. Sodium, also found in table salt, may increase blood pressure, especially for people who are salt sensitive.

To help prevent high blood pressure, it's a good idea to watch your sodium intake. On average, North American adults consume roughly

---

A Note from Dr. Jonas
WATCH OUT FOR MSG

For an estimated 2 percent of the population, the small amount of MSG Chinese chefs often use to flavor Chinese dishes may be enough to induce MSG symptom complex, a reaction characterized by a burning sensation at the back of the neck, dizziness, nausea, headache, or breathing difficulties. Symptoms may last for up to an hour. If you're not sensitive to MSG and don't need to restrict sodium, MSG won't do you any harm. If you suspect that you're sensitive to MSG, however, skip the unpleasantness and ask your server to tell the chef to refrain from using MSG on your order.

3,000 milligrams of sodium per person each day (1 ½ teaspoons of salt). The good news? That's just 600 milligrams (¼ teaspoon) more than the limit of 2,400 daily milligrams of sodium recommended by the American Heart Association.

Still, consider flavoring foods with lemon juice and other seasonings instead of salt, or opt for low-sodium soy sauce, which has half the sodium of regular soy sauce. Also, eat fewer ready-to-eat foods. Salt lurks in canned and instant soups, condiments such as mustard and ketchup, frozen dinners, macaroni and cheese from the box, canned chili with beans, chicken bouillon cubes, ready-made pasta sauce, pretzels, and pickles. To choose wisely, read food labels and choose canned and other processed foods with a Daily Value (DV) for sodium of no more than 5 percent.

—————— GLOBAL EATING SECRET #14 ——————

Establish a Healthy Routine

While diet counts for a lot, to stay healthy for the long haul, study after study shows that it takes more than diet. We're all the sum of our parts, and what we eat is only one component of our health profile. Physical activity, environmental and other stresses, genes, and the social fabric of our lives all contribute to our healthiness or the lack of it.

The Chinese seem to have a grasp on the big picture of health. It has been said about the Chinese that their habits tend to be very regular. "They go to bed at a certain time and get up at a certain time and they take naps. They eat at certain times and they don't snack," observes Georgia Guldan.

While it's politically incorrect and dangerous to generalize, studies show that people who are conscientious about their health habits and who are not always seeking instant gratification—those who don't "act now and worry about the consequences later"—tend to live longer. This way of living may not appeal to you, but when it comes to health habits, it may pay to err on the safe side.

Chinese Dietary Guidelines

By now, you probably have the U.S. dietary guidelines memorized: Eat a variety of foods; maintain a healthy weight; choose a diet low in fat, saturated fat, and cholesterol; choose a diet with plenty of vegetables, fruits, and grain products; use sugars, salt and sodium, and alcohol only in moderation. "Everything in moderation" is this diet plan's motto. But these kinds of messages aren't exclusive to North America. Many countries develop dietary guidelines. Here are those the Chinese government created to point its populace to better health.

1 Eat a variety of foods.
2 Eat foods in reasonable amounts.
3 Select some less refined grains.
4 Eat a moderate amount of fat and oil.
5 Limit the amount of salt eaten.
6 Eat few sweets.
7 Drink alcohol in moderation.
8 Allocate the three meals reasonably evenly. (Source: The Chinese Nutrition Society, "Dietary Guidelines for the Chinese," *Acta Nutrimenta Sinica* 12(3):10–12.)

4

FRANCE
The Good Life Savored

To safeguard one's health at the cost of too strict a diet is a tiresome illness indeed.

—François Duc de La Rochefoucauld (1613–1680), French writer and moralist

Flaky croissants, snails and frogs' legs swimming in garlic butter, triple-cream *fromage* (cheese), melt-in-your-mouth foie gras (goose or duck liver), terrines of pâtés, crème caramel, clouds of chocolate mousse—the list goes on. In the northern and central regions of France, including Île-de-France (Paris) and Normandy, these and other specialties made with butter and cream and other animal fats are featured on countless menus. All will invariably make your taste buds sing. Eating well is an integral part of the national heritage of the whole of France, but mind you, not everyone in France is a natural-born chef. Restaurant eating, however, is another thing entirely. In the smallest *ferme-auberge* (farm inn) or the most formal urban bistro, you can count on French fare that will be lovingly prepared with the exactitude of a surgeon.

To say the French know their food is an understatement. It has been said that even French children are serious gourmands, with their expanded palates and their weekday two-hour multicourse lunches (the norm throughout France). Doubtless, such a lunch is an integral part of their education.

For North Americans, a visit to France can be puzzling. By just glancing in the window of a *pâtisserie* showcasing dozens of artfully coifed French *gâteaux* (cakes) and pastries, or a *fromagerie* (cheese shop), you can almost feel your arteries slamming shut and the pounds creeping on. Surely the French, especially those residing in the butter-loving central and northern regions, are paying the price for their daily indulgences. You would think that being overweight is a national problem in France and trying to slim down, a societal obsession—even more so than it is in North America. But as you may know from all that has been written about the French Paradox, quite the opposite is true. Oddly enough, the French, despite their attachment to the finer foods in life, are some of the healthiest and perhaps guilt-free people on the planet.

France at a Glance

Moderate drinking

- Chronic excess drinking is never healthy; the French are masters of the art of drinking in moderation. Their tempered one-to-two-drink-a-day habit may be what's keeping their hearts healthier despite their traditional high-fat diet. Studies show that wine and alcohol itself may contain antioxidants that raise levels of "good" HDL cholesterol, the kind that prevents fatty deposits from building up on artery walls. A diet that contains moderate amounts of alcohol may also reduce the risk of stroke by as much as 50 percent by preventing blood clots from forming. An added bonus: Moderate drinking has also been shown to boost longevity.

Lots of fruits and vegetables

- Even though the typical French diet is high in fat (35 to 38 percent of total calories), the French also eat, on average, four or more servings of vegetables a day—perhaps another clue to why their rates of heart disease and some cancers are less than in the United States.

No snacking or dieting

- The French traditionally don't snack, and many also eat their largest meal in the middle of the day—two reasons why the French may be leaner despite their high-fat diet.

- Dieting in France is rarely taken to the extreme. Prepackaged meals and other U.S.-style "diet" foods are considered an insult to their sophisticated palates. Instead, when the French are watching their weight, many make small changes here and there, like declining the cheese course or eating their baguette sans butter.

Staying Healthy the French Way

Consider these facts:

- The French diet is high in saturated fat—35 to 38 percent of total calories come from fat—compared to 34 percent in North America. In fact, the U.S. dietary recommendation to get less than 30 percent of your total calories from fat is very un-French. According to one study involving 837 French participants, only 14 percent derived less than 30 percent of their energy from fat, and only 4 percent derived less than 10 percent of their energy from saturated fat. As you know, a high-fat diet has been associated with the increased incidence of cardiovascular disease and different forms of cancer.

- Collectively, the "good" heart-protective HDL cholesterol levels and rates of hypertension (high blood pressure) in the French are about the same as they are in North Americans, but the total serum cholesterol levels are higher in the French.

- And like the citizens of Mediterranean countries and the United States, many French also smoke cigarettes, a well-known risk factor for heart disease and cancer.

Tally the score and the French come out the loser. "If you look at all of their risk factors, you'd predict that the French would have at least 50 percent more heart attacks than we do," says R. Curtis Ellison, M.D., a medical researcher at the Boston University School of Medicine who has studied the French Paradox extensively.

But quite the opposite is true. Compared with North Americans, for example, the French are much less likely to die of heart disease. According to the American Heart Association, out of thirty-five selected countries, France reports death rates from cardiovascular diseases that are among the lowest in the world—second only to Japan. The prevalence of heart disease in northern and central France is said to resemble that of the Mediterranean countries, where the proportion of saturated fat in the diet is much lower.

Moreover, besides keeping hearts healthier despite the permissive diet, the French are also better at combating cancer. For example, they report incidence rates of breast cancer that are 50 percent lower, on average, than in the United States. Also, their incidence rates of colon and prostate cancers are roughly 30 and 60 percent lower, respectively, than those in the United

Food for Thought

By 2050, it's projected that 150,000 centenarians (those making it to age 100) will be living in France, a 750-fold increase since 1950.

Food for Thought

When it comes to food, the French can be set in their codified ways. Order a coffee-ice-cream-with-chocolate-sauce sundae at an ice cream shop in Paris, for example, where standard vanilla-chocolate or vanilla-strawberry sundaes are the norm, and you're likely to be refused because that combination "doesn't taste good." A general rule when it comes to eating in France: The French know food (although they can be wrong). Nonetheless, when you're on their turf, let them take care of you.

States. When matched up against France, the United States reports a more than 60 percent higher incidence of all cancers.

A further injustice: In spite of their hedonistic ways, the French are leaner. Eight percent of the French now qualify as obese, which has many French epidemiologists concerned. Still, the French lag far behind most other industrialized countries; for example, in the United States, roughly 22 percent of the population has a body mass index (BMI) of 30 or more, an increase from 13 percent in 1960. (Knowing your BMI, the gold standard for assessing obesity in populations and in scientific studies, is one important way to keep tabs on your health.) And on average, the French live longer than North Americans: French men, by about a year; French women, by two and one-half years.

How much of all of this is in the genes? Probably not much. Case in point: When the French move to Montreal and begin to consume a more U.S.-style diet, "they get fatter," says Dr. Ellison, and their heart disease rates begin to resemble that of North Americans.

French Diet Secrets Revealed

How do the French do it? What can we discover from the French diet that will enhance our health and longevity? Researchers have been asking these questions for years and have only recently begun to develop useful answers from the dozens of cross-cultural studies that have been conducted.

In the beginning, the French Paradox was linked to olive oil consumption (although butter, not olive oil, prevails in the heart-healthy regions of central and northern France), the rich foie gras French farmers have been producing for centuries by methodically fattening their birds, and the wine the French customarily sip with meals. Indeed, researchers have speculated that some of the answers to the mysteries of the longevity and the healthfulness of the French may lie in their intake of particular foods. More recent studies point to the overall quality of the diet and the long-standing culinary traditions the French stubbornly hold on to, despite the U.S.-style fast-food chains that have been infecting the scene in major gastronomy centers like Paris and Lyon.

As countless studies have shown, your diet can make *la différence* in helping you to reduce your risk of developing a major chronic killer such as heart disease or cancer, and to keep your weight in check. This chapter reveals many of the French diet secrets that can help you stay healthy and slim—secrets that have withstood the test of time and the scrutiny of scientific testing and observation.

Go Ahead, Raise Your Glass of Wine, but Not Too Often

Role models in winemaking the world over, the French have been producing fine wines in the Bordeaux, Burgundy, Rhône, and Champagne regions since pre-Roman times. Consequently, wine doesn't carry with it the big-deal status that many Americans reserve for it. "Wine is a part of life and a part of food. You can't have a great meal without a great wine," states Annie Jacquet-Bentley, a Parisian restaurant and marketing consultant in Birchrunville, Pennsylvania, who runs L'École des Chefs, a one-on-one internship program that ushers Americans into the exclusive world of Paris's top restaurants. Jacquet-Bentley is echoing a common French sentiment regarding wine's important though nonchalant role at mealtime; the French typically sip a glass or two of wine at dinner, perhaps even at lunch, a habit that is suspected to counteract many of the ill effects of a high-fat diet.

Wine consumption in France has been falling in recent years due to its sagging popularity among younger generations, but according to the Wine Institute in San Francisco, the French still imbibe more than 900,000 gallons of wine annually, which is nearly double U.S. consumption. "The French never go a long time without alcohol," concludes Boston University medical researcher R. Curtis Ellison, M.D. That may be one of the reasons for their healthier hearts.

The Health Benefits of *Moderate* Drinking

The health benefits of wine and alcohol in general have long been the subject of spirited research. *"À votre santé"* (To your health) is more than a tasteful toast. At last count, there are at least twenty-five different mechanisms by which alcohol consumption, in moderation to be sure, can lower the risk of heart disease, Dr. Ellison estimates. For example, studies suggest that moderate alcohol consumption—one to two modest-size glasses a day, the amount many French people typically consume regularly—may raise blood serum levels of "good" HDL cholesterol, the kind that prevents fatty deposits from building up on artery walls. Other studies suggest that *moderate* drinking—

defined as 12 ounces of beer, 4 to 5 ounces of wine, or 1.5 ounces of 80-proof liquor per day, all of which supply about half an ounce of pure alcohol—may reduce the risk of stroke by as much as 50 percent by acting on platelets in the blood to prevent clots from forming.

Furthermore, for reasons yet to be determined, if you choose to drink, light drinking may also help you live longer. According to an observational study published in the *New England Journal of Medicine* in 1997 that involved 490,000 participants, the rates of death from all cardiovascular diseases were 30 to 40 percent lower for the men and women who consumed at least one glass of spirits daily. The study reports 20 percent lower rates of death from all causes among participants who drank one glass a day, compared to those who abstained.

Previously, researchers attributed these cardiovascular benefits to the wine drinking exclusively, specifically citing the antioxidants and phytochemicals wine contains. But now that thinking has changed. "At least 60 percent of the protection you get from drinking comes from the alcohol itself," Dr. Ellison estimates. According to studies, you can get antioxidant benefits from drinking grape juice, but you'll get only one-third as much as you would if you drank the alcoholic version. The fermentation associated with alcohol formation increases a beverage's disease-fighting antioxidant content.

The French Alcohol-Cancer Connection

You may have heard that drinking moderate quantities of red wine, in particular, can not only help fight heart disease but also help prevent cancer. The secret ingredients include resveratrol and other antioxidants called polyphenols found in grape skins, which may block the action of carcinogens, inhibit tumor growth, and cause precancerous cells to revert to normal. Alcohol, however, has a dual personality: Consumed in moderation, it may protect your heart; but in excess, it has also been shown to be a carcinogen. A review reported in the *Journal of the American Medical Association,* for example, analyzed six studies on the relationship between alcohol and breast cancer. It concluded that women who regularly consume two to five drinks a day increase their risk of breast cancer by more than 40 percent. According to the National Cancer Institute, there's also a strong association between excess alcohol intake and cancers of the mouth, pharynx, esophagus, and larynx. (This risk is compounded if you're a smoker.) Excessive alcohol consumption may also increase your risk of colorectal (colon and rectal) cancer, according to a major report from the American Institute for Cancer Research (AICR), a nonprofit educational organization in Washington, D.C., which analyzed 4,500 research studies.

There's more. *Chronic excess drinking* may also increase the risk of stroke, osteoporosis, liver damage, creeping blood pressure, infertility, accidents, premenstrual syndrome, and insomnia. The French, in particular, suffer higher rates of cirrhosis of the liver and other liver diseases than do North Americans, because a certain percentage of the French population takes drinking too far. It's not uncommon on your morning walk to work in Paris, for example, to see patrons at neighborhood cafés lingering over a glass of wine.

The Key Is Moderation

To reduce your risk of heart disease without increasing your cancer risk, play it safe. If you choose to drink, it pays to put the brakes on. Men are advised to consume no more than two drinks a day, and women should stop at one—the levels shown by research to protect against heart disease. (Remember, one drink equals 12 ounces of beer, 4 to 5 ounces of wine, or one 1.5-ounce shot of 80-proof liquor per day, all of which supply about 0.5 ounce of pure alcohol.) Whether you choose to drink in moderation or abstain, be sure to get plenty of exercise, lose weight if you need to, and eat fewer foods high in saturated fat, such as red meat and full-fat dairy products, to reduce your overall risk of heart disease.

To keep drinking within the boundaries of one to two glasses a day, develop a strategy: Think of alcohol like food. The same rules apply. For example, just as it's smarter to dole yourself one or two cookies (or your contraband of choice) at a time instead of sitting down with the whole box, it's a good idea to avoid ordering wine by the bottle when you're eating out with others. Go with a glass instead. At home, serve yourself wine by the half bottle, shared with others. On days you don't drink, do as the French do and serve yourself Perrier or a favorite nonalcoholic beverage in a special glass. As

---

A Note from Dr. Jonas
WOMEN AND ALCOHOL

Alcohol packs a bigger punch in women. One drink in a woman is generally equal to two drinks in a man; as a result, women get drunk faster than men and may suffer alcohol's negative long-term effects sooner. That's because women are typically smaller than men and have less body mass. They also have a higher proportion of body fat, and have less fluid in their bodies to dilute alcohol. Furthermore, women also have less of a liver enzyme called alcohol dehydrogenase, which helps the body purge itself of alcohol. For all these reasons, equivalent doses of alcohol become more concentrated in a woman's body more quickly. The two-for-one disparity women experience, however, levels off after menopause, when the amount of alcohol dehydrogenase in men's and women's bodies equalizes.

A Note from Dr. Jonas
ALCOHOL AND FOLIC ACID

Alcohol blunts the absorption of folate, the food form of folic acid, a B vitamin especially important for women of childbearing age. Even just one drink a day can make this nutrient dent in your diet. To reduce this damage from alcohol, it's especially advisable for women to take a vitamin supplement that contains folic acid before or after having a few drinks. By taking a daily folic acid supplement, women may also reduce their colon cancer risk over the long run. According to the results of the Nurses' Health Study published in the *Annals of Internal Medicine* in 1998, which involved nearly 90,000 women over a fourteen-year period, those who took folic acid supplements, whose intakes exceeded 400 micrograms (mcg) per day, were more than 30 percent less likely to develop colon cancer than those who consumed only 200 mcg or less per day of the B vitamin.

the French are well aware, the accoutrements of drinking are a legitimate part of the enjoyment.

Drink Only with Food

Something the French rarely do is drink without eating. (In France, even wineshops—*troquets*—serve food.) The common habit of winding down at the end of the day with a drink is not part of their culture, which may be another reason why they stay so slim on a diet that welcomes wine. When you start out on empty, ethanol—the intoxicating agent in alcoholic beverages—makes a beeline for your brain. Alcohol zones in on the frontal lobe, the judgment and reasoning center, to tinker with your resolve to not overeat. Those potato chips you've been resisting? Forget it! After a round or two of drinks on empty, you could then find yourself polishing off half the bowl, with dip on your lip to prove it.

To curb the craving, pace yourself. If you're at a party, open the evening with seltzer mixed with fruit juice or a virgin Bloody Mary and nosh on some low-fat crackers, a smidgen of cheese, and some carrot sticks. Then go ahead and have a glass of the real thing. (Or, better yet, *à la française*, wait to drink until dinner.) Either way, by the time you have your first drink, you'll have a culinary cushion to delay the rate that alcohol rushes to your brain to toil with your good diet intentions.

GLOBAL EATING SECRET #16

Make Lunch a Megameal

With their love of rich pâtés, buttery cheeses, and flaky pastries, the French are a walking enigma. Why isn't the battle with obesity and overweight in France more intense than it is in North America? As mentioned earlier, the French have less than half the rate of obesity than exists in the United States.

"You rarely see a fat person in France," many a tourist has uttered, upon recounting their recent stroll down the Avenue des Champs-Élysées, the famous grand thoroughfare in Paris that showcases historic buildings, museums, galleries, churches, shops, gardens, and U.S.-style fast-food restaurants as manicured as the French who walk the avenue daily. According to government statistics, the French consume roughly the same amount of calories daily as does the typical North American. (But don't think it's the French themselves who are keeping track. France has few get-out-the-calculator calorie counters.) While the rates of obesity in France are ever so gradually creeping upward, the universal question remains: How do the French, in spite of their seemingly hedonistic approach to eating, keep their amazing figures?

Lunch the French Way

One clue to their relative leanness may be found in their meal patterns. A major difference between North Americans and the French is that the French don't take lunch lightly. Traditionally, as any guidebook will tell you, the noon meal in France is a major one, especially in the rural areas. To illustrate this point, in the early 1990s, Dr. Ellison conducted a study comparing the lifestyles of fifty Americans living in a Boston suburb with the lifestyles of fifty Parisians in an attempt to clarify the differences between the two cultures. Dr. Ellison found that by 2:00 P.M. each day, the French had consumed 60 percent of their daily calories. This major calorie load typically lasted them another six hours, when they'd sit down for their evening meal at around 8:00 P.M. Conversely, the Americans in this study took in only 40 percent of their calories by 2:00 P.M., had a snack several hours later, and saved their largest meal for dinner. They spent the rest of the evening engaged in sedentary activities such as watching TV. In effect, they were consuming the majority of their calorie load when they least needed it and had less chance to burn it off.

Traditionally, the French have allocated one to two hours of their workday for lunch. (On Sunday, however, lunch can last three to four hours; you may still be sitting at the table at four or five o'clock.) In rural areas, lunch—

Food for Thought

Don't let the pâtisseries (pastry shops) throughout France selling such delights as gorgeous cakes and luscious napoleons fool you. Many French don't eat these rich desserts every day. Rather, they tend to reserve such treats for Sundays and special occasions. What's most often served after dinner during the week? Fruit that is eaten with a fork and knife, such as poached pears or prunes stewed in wine.

A Note from Dr. Jonas
ARE YOU AN END-OF-DAY EATER?

Watch out. It's a pattern that could lead to weight gain and/or difficulty losing weight, especially if you then indulge in a snack or two close to bedtime. Studies have shown that when people eat just before going to bed, their body temperature rises less than when they eat the same food and stay awake. This suggests that if you eat before going to sleep, your body may conserve rather than burn most of the extra calories.

Food for Thought

North Americans do breakfast better than the French. Typically, the French fuel their mornings with coffee or café au lait and a piece of baguette with jam. A breakfast of whole-grain cereal with low-fat or skim milk and fruit or fruit juice (minus the bacon and eggs, of course), which is enjoyed by an increasing number of North Americans, is far healthier than the French version.

even on weekdays—is akin to a sacred ritual and is a time for the family to gather. "If you come into a small town in France around noon, you won't see anyone. But you'll hear this incredible clinking of silverware and pots and pans through the shuttered windows, and the conversation going on in the house," says Lynn Kutner, a New Yorker who has spent summers since 1971 with her family in a charming village perched in the hills near Cannes. On the other hand, unless the French are eating out, dinner is traditionally downplayed. Though it's graciously served, dinner at home in France on a weekday is typically a relatively minor meal.

Elongating Your Lunch "Hour"

The megameal at noon is gradually fading in France's urban areas. But the French haven't totally given up their time-honored structured mealtimes. The North American habit of speed eating, which is a good way to take in loads of calories without even realizing it, has yet to make its way to France. A rare sight in France is someone eating while driving or walking, or eating while negotiating the foot traffic. The habit of, say, grabbing a carton of yogurt and eating at one's desk, or skipping lunch altogether and wrestling sustenance from the vending machine when hunger calls, is also frowned upon.

Unlike the culinary traditions of countries such as Japan, where they're eager to adapt the latest food trend to make it uniquely Japanese, the culinary traditions of France die hard. We're told that even if the French don't have a lot of time, they will often sit down and have some variation of the standard two- or three-course meal at lunch—for example, a sandwich and a salad or crudité (raw fruit or vegetables), or a small steak with *pommes frites* (yes, french fries) followed by a salad. To opt for a lunch like this, which may or may not include wine, you're likely to go to a café or *brasserie* (a large café that serves quick meals).

Who has time for a midday meal even to this extent? Not you? It's still possible that you can make more of this much underrated eating opportunity so you'll have a chance to take in and burn a significant calorie load during the day, when your body and your brain most need it. Make a point to escape from your office and squeeze in twenty to thirty minutes to refuel and take a breather. Or, plan ahead and bring a substantial lunch from home. To get the maximum satisfaction out of each mouthful, however, be sure to ditch your desk. Try to honor your lunch hour and only eat in "designated eating places," such as at your kitchen table, in the cafeteria at your office, or in a restaurant.

Curtail Snacking

According to the Calorie Control Council, 43 percent of dieters in the United States say that snacking too much is the reason they haven't maintained their desired weight. Unlike North Americans, who typically consume as many as three snacks a day—more than 20 percent of a day's total calories—the French don't usually partake in this between-meal ritual. This non-habit may contribute to the comparatively higher proportion of slimmer figures found in France.

French children may have an after-school *goûter* (snack)—often a croissant or *pain au chocolat* (a boxy croissant with a hidden melted dollop of dark chocolate)—to tide them over until dinner, but regular snacking just isn't part of the adult French culture. Their substantial lunch often usurps the need for an afternoon snack. And because the demand for snacks in France isn't as great as it is in the United States, the snack food industry isn't yet in full force. Snacks are a novelty and priced accordingly. A small bag of potato chips, for example, can run $2 to $3.

A Note from Dr. Jonas
THE ROAD TO A HEALTHY DIET IS A PERSONAL PATH

When it comes to eating healthier, there's no single, absolute, standard definition of success. As I mentioned earlier, you need to set personal, realistic goals that align with your capabilities and your lifestyle. Let's say you've decided to give up fatty takeout dinners but don't have time to cook—what are you going to eat? Make sure you stock your kitchen with low-fat frozen meals, bagged salads, and veggies each week so you have easy, healthy options on hand. In other words, we can often set ourselves up for success over time if we plan right. While you're developing your goals for eating healthier, troubleshoot now so you can design a plan that's truly doable. And keep in mind that the diet and health "secrets" offered throughout this book are only starting points. Feel free to customize them to fit your objectives and your lifestyle.

A Snack-Attack Culture

According to the Snack Food Association, the commercial snack food industry took root in North America as far back as 1853 when potato chips (then called "crunch potato slices") were whimsically invented at a resort in Saratoga, New York. Since then, snacking has become so common that it's difficult to tell North Americans to give up this timeworn habit. But snacking may be getting out of hand.

During the past two decades, North Americans' snack food consumption has increased 200 percent, and has even threatened to replace breakfast, lunch, and/or dinner for many of us. Chocolate, potato chips, and other popular high-fat items continue to be popular sellers in this multi-billion-dollar industry. According to a 1996 survey by Roper Starch Worldwide, Inc., most North Americans no longer eat three meals a day. (Just one in four eats breakfast, lunch, and dinner, and nothing else on a typical day—down from 33 percent in 1985.) This has increased our reliance on snacks.

Don't misunderstand. Snacks, if chosen judiciously, can be good for you. Many snacks in the dairy, whole grain, and produce categories, for example, such as nonfat yogurt, instant lentil soup, and pears and berries, offer complex carbohydrates, an important energy source, as well as calcium, iron, and fiber, three important nutrients many North Americans' diets especially lack. For many of us, however, snack foods—the usual suspects—present an invitation for weight gain.

For some time, in newspapers and consumer magazines, nutritionists have been telling consumers that snacking could actually help us lose weight by saving us from getting too hungry and then overeating at the next meal. But recent research suggests that this isn't true. In fact, snacking is likely to be fattening. According to a study conducted by the Department of Internal Medicine and Nutrition at the Hôtel-Dieu in Paris that involved 273 obese French women, 60 percent of whom snacked, snacking increased total calorie consumption. Those who snacked also ate more at and between meals.

This study supports the emerging theory that the amount you eat between meals increases, rather than diminishes, your total calorie intake for the day. "If you eat a snack midmorning or midafternoon, it has no effect on what you're going to eat for lunch or dinner," says David Levitsky, Ph.D., professor of nutrition and psychology at Cornell University. "We don't decrease our food intake at subsequent meals by snacking."

For many of us, the desire to snack is often more environmental than biological. In general, if we see it, we'll eat it. And the more frequently we snack, the higher our total calorie intake will be, says Levitsky. To reduce your calorie load and keep your weight in check, do like the French: Snack less, if at all.

Attention Snackaholics: Negotiating the Vending Machine

It's three hours until lunch and you feel light-headed; your stomach's churning. You can't concentrate. What to do? Don't feel guilty if you must snack. It's okay occasionally. Your best bet is to plan snacks that are low in fat and calories. It happens that healthier choices are now available at many vending machines. But many offerings can still be high-fat, high-calorie snacks that can sabotage your best intentions. (Even the so-called healthy snacks such as low-fat cookies or crackers can be high in sugar and calories and low in fiber, a combination that may leave you hankering for more.) Instead of falling victim to the vending machine when the midafternoon munchies hit, plan ahead. Healthy, satisfying foods to keep around your home and your office include low-calorie beverages such as herbal tea or flavored sparkling water; nonfat yogurt (if a refrigerator is available); apples, oranges, or bananas; small bags of rice cakes; tiny boxes of raisins or animal crackers; packets of instant oatmeal or diet hot chocolate mix.

If you have trouble stopping at one, keep these snacks at home and bring in a single snack daily. If you find yourself in front of the vending machine anyway, hold off on pressing the button for a candy bar or a bag of Doritos. First, have something to drink—water or a diet beverage—which might just fill you up. Registered dietitians tell us that the air in office buildings can be dry and dehydrating; you may think you're hungry when you're actually thirsty. If you can't resist, do yourself a favor. Don't guiltily devour those potato chips or that chocolate bar. *A la française,* s-a-v-o-r one portion very slowly. Set a timer and challenge yourself to finish the bag or the bar in no less than ten minutes, suggests Dan Stettner, Ph.D., director of psychology in the department of preventive and nutritional medicine at the William Beaumont Hospital Center in Birmingham, Michigan. The slower you eat a snack, or a regular meal for that matter, the more likely you are to feel satisfied with just one moderate-size portion.

——— G L O B A L   E A T I N G   S E C R E T   #18 ———

Savor Variety

Bigger house. Bigger car. Bigger restaurant meals. The more-is-better-phenomenon we've come to expect in North America is positively foreign to the French. Take restaurant meals. One Parisian who spends part of the year in the United States and frequently entertains French friends and relatives who visit here, says that "when the French come to the United States, they're appalled at the quantity of food served in the restaurants." At French restaurants in France, you're apt to get a chicken breast or a leg, for example, not a whole, a half, or even a quarter chicken for a main course. Moreover, the French find the idea of taking home dinner leftovers comical. "There is no such thing as a doggy bag in France because they don't ever give you enough to put anything in it," joked another Parisian interviewed during the course of research for this book.

Clean Your Plate

Why are the portions in France so small? In short, during the first half of the twentieth century, a depressed economy as well as inflation, widespread unemployment, and profound social unrest wrought by two world wars took a toll on the food supply in France. In many cases, food was scarce; in others, nonexistent. Today, as a result, you'll still hear French parents telling their children to clean their plates, a reprimand that has been passed down through the generations. Small portions are perhaps a backlash against the national abhorrence to food waste that the French have developed throughout their history. And according to the World Health Organization's *Comparative Analysis of Nutrition Policies in WHO European Member States,* France is keenly "aware of large amounts of food being destroyed and dumped due to EU (European Union) policies instead of being distributed to the needy."

Despite the modest portions, however, don't think the French are walking away from the table hungry. Their portions may be diminutive compared to ours, but the French make up for it by eating more courses—even at the meals they have at home. On the dinner menu, for example, a first course might be a small, artfully crafted plate of crudités (raw vegetables), followed by a main course of tournedos (small fillets of beef) with a little side of *frites* (fried potatoes) and vegetables, such as asparagus. And always, you can expect a baguette of heavenly bread, the quality of which is difficult to match outside of France. Then, for the cheese course, which is always an event in which one to four well-chosen cheeses are presented and judiciously consumed, you'll take just one or two artfully apportioned pieces. (French women who are watching their weight may choose to abstain from the course entirely. They may also neglect to butter their baguette, but you won't notice since they're not apt to make their weight-loss strategy a topic of discussion. And forget diet drinks like SlimFast or special packaged low-calorie meals. Passing on the cheese and the butter is about as extreme as the French get when it comes to dieting.) A salad, which is usually only dressed greens such as curly endive, butter lettuce, radicchio, or arugula, might also be served with the cheese course. For the finale, as mentioned earlier, there will be a piece of fruit. If it's a special occasion or a Sunday, however, a selection of those famous French pastries may be presented.

Compared to the megasize portions now being served in many North American restaurants, the standard portions served in French restaurants look like airline food. Still, it's okay to eat some meals the North American way (larger portions, fewer courses) as long as you're aware of how much you're eating and are willing to make changes at your next meal, such as eating a bit less. The key: Learn to recognize a standard serving size. The chart below, which is based on USDA dietary guidelines, can help you to size up your servings and right-size your mental image of foods at mealtime.

Right-sizing *Your* Servings

FOOD GROUP	FOOD	RECOMMENDED SERVING SIZE	THINK:
Bread, cereal, rice, & pasta	Pasta, rice, ready-to-eat or cooked cereal	½ cup	Your fist
	Bagel	½	Your palm
	Roll, biscuit, or muffin	1 "small"	Standard lightbulb
Fruit	Fresh fruit	1 "medium"	Baseball
Vegetable	Potatoes	1 "medium" russet	Business card
	Raw or cooked vegetables	½ cup	Ice cream scoop
Meat, poultry, fish	Lean meat, poultry, or fish	2 to 3 ounces	Computer mouse
Milk, yogurt, & cheese	Skim milk or nonfat yogurt	1 cup	Regulation takeout coffee cup
	Lowfat cheese	1 ounce	Pair of dice
Fats, oils, & sweets	Margarine, vegetable oil, or mayonnaise	1 teaspoon	A quarter ($)
	Diet margarine or reduced-calorie mayonnaise	1 tablespoon	Triple-size cotton ball (cosmetic cotton ball)
	Regular salad dressing	2 tablespoons	2 tea bags
	French fries	10	Pen cap (one fry)
	Piece of cake	3" × 3" piece	Post-it note

Health Is in the Structure

Serving meals in courses tends to formalize and lengthen the French eating experience. It also ensures that the French diet is varied, which helps the French counteract the effects of a comparatively high intake of saturated fat. During a French meal, one by one, nearly every food group, especially fruits and vegetables, is represented, which may also help explain the French Paradox. Even though the French diet is high in fat, its also hits the USDA dietary guideline on the mark—choose a diet with plenty of grain products, vegetables, and fruit. According to a study that assessed the quality of the French diet, close to 90 percent of the 837 French participants scored a maximum of 5 points in the category of "dietary diversity," the number of major food groups consumed daily. In this study, the average repertoire of "core" foods in the French diet was roughly thirty items. In comparison, only 33 percent of American adults scored this well in food consumption studies.

Like the French, many North Americans consume a diet that's high in saturated fat, but unlike the French, many of us still don't consume enough fruits and vegetables to counteract its ill effects. According to the USDA Continuing Survey of Food Intakes by Individuals, we need to focus on having a lower consumption of saturated fat and a higher consumption of fruit.

A simple change, such as eating the recommended five servings of fruits and vegetables each day, would prevent 20 percent or more of all cases of cancer, states the American Institute for Cancer Research, a nonprofit educational organization in Washington, D.C. Couple that dietary change with not smoking, and you may have the potential to reduce your cancer risk by 60 to 70 percent.

Eating generous and frequent servings of fruits and vegetables may also reduce your risk of heart disease in the presence of a high-fat diet. (Although it's still a good idea to try to reduce your total fat intake to 30 percent of total calories or less. This guideline applies to your

---

A Note from Dr. Jonas
DIVERSIFYING YOUR DIET

Of course, "eat a variety of foods" is one of the dietary guidelines. Yeah, yeah, yeah, you're probably saying to yourself. It sounds vaguely like your mother telling you to clean your plate. But there's solid science supporting this mandate. The most impressive research on disease prevention suggests that it's not enough, for example, to just eat your broccoli. You've also got to eat spinach, potatoes, oranges, whole grains, beans, and low-fat dairy products. Every food and food group, especially the fruit and vegetable group, offers a profile of disease-fighting substances such as antioxidants, phytochemicals, and fiber as different as your DNA is from your neighbor's. Researchers believe these disease warriors work together as a team to defend your body against major threats like cancer, heart disease, and osteoporosis—the principal reason why a varied diet rich in plant foods is so important for good health over the long run.

total fat intake over a week, not to any one food.) A 1993 study pitting France against Finland, for example, where the death rates from coronary heart disease were four to five times higher, concluded that France, where people consumed more plant foods, including small amounts of liquid vegetable oils and more vegetables (and thus more antioxidants), had lower rates of death from coronary heart disease despite a high-saturated-fat diet. In the study, French participants consumed four times more vegetables than the Finns—about four to five servings a day—and three and half times less milk and butterfat.

Don't Feel Guilty about Food

Another clue to the leanness of the French is the absence of a love-hate relationship with food. Dieting in general is seldom a topic for open discussion. "Food is a life pleasure and it's meant to be enjoyed," says Annie Jacquet-Bentley, a Parisian restaurant consultant. The French aren't afraid of rich sauces. They're not worried about eating the skin of their roasted chicken. "If you eat too much, the next day you eat less. But you don't punish yourself," says Jacquet-Bentley. "It's better to be consistent."

Indeed, for years, health professionals in the media have been counseling North Americans about diet guilt and why it's important to avoid catastrophizing if they overeat. A common scenario: You eat more than you planned, then figure, "I've really blown it, so I might as well give up for today and start over tomorrow." Trouble is, often you don't start over tomorrow. Or you do, and you simply repeat the pattern. That's when guilt—the biggest motivation killer of all—sets in and you're sunk. Along with the guilt, feelings of dieting failure can take control, which can lead to not only dropping the low-fat approach but bingeing as well.

To release yourself from this emotional roller coaster, do as the French do and isolate the event. Say, "Okay, I just had the cheese soufflé, and a baguette with butter, and the chocolate cake. Now, I'll go back to my regular routine." What the French seem to understand (that we often don't) is that in the long run, it's normal rather than harmful to slip now and then.

——— G L O B A L   E A T I N G   S E C R E T   #19 ———
Take the Time to Cook Properly

In North America, we're enamored with food that can be zapped. When the going gets tough, the tough pick up the can opener or reach for the frozen,

Food for Thought

It's typically French to eat your salad after, not before, your entrée. And because portions are modest, you'll have room. "The salad helps fill you up," one French friend explained. But if you're trying to lose weight, actually eating your greens before the entrée might be better. The logic: Having salad first helps curb your appetite so you'll be less likely to down a second helping of a more calorie-laden dish later on in the meal. By the way, the French almost never douse their greens with sweet, saturated-fat-filled salad dressings like we're known to do. Bleu cheese and French salad dressing are not at all French. On the French table, vinaigrette, a standard olive oil-vinegar-mustard combination, is the rule.

microwave meal. It seems that everyone wants a great meal on the table in ten minutes or less, and we'll gladly take any shortcut to save time and effort.

Enter the French. Although more French are in a hurry these days, they're still famously fastidious about their food and seldom think of preparing a meal without using only the freshest, highest-quality ingredients, which also happen to have the greater nutrient value. To cut corners, rather than buy something that's already prepared or canned, they're more apt to use a fresh product that's partially prepped, such as carrots that have been grated, beets that have already been cooked, or peeled potatoes. But the meal they put together is a work of their own, so they know exactly what they're putting into their bodies and exactly what they're serving their family.

Health-Promoting Meals Start with Fresh, Quality Ingredients

Because of this concern for quality and freshness, which maximizes flavor and dining enjoyment, the French tend to eat closer to the land. For example, when you buy a chicken from a local French butcher, it may still have its head, feet, and entrails; only after you've chosen it does the butcher clean it for you. The chicken will also likely be hormone free. It may also have a large label with a serial number that can help you trace where it was raised and killed, if you need to.

Similarly, most French wouldn't dream of buying a frozen baguette, although they are available. Instead, they're likely to pick up a freshly baked one for lunch at a local *boulangerie* (bakery), and another one later in the day for dinner. They're also known to inspect their produce, which they might buy at a local farm-

---

A Note from Dr. Jonas
FIGHTING THE FEAR OF FAILURE

As you may know, trying to eat healthier and actually doing it are two different things. What holds many of us back from even trying, however, is the "fear-of-failure" state of mind, the all-time motivation killer. You know you suffer from this mental malady if you find yourself saying things like, "I can't lose weight, so why try?" Or, "I've tried changing my diet, but it's no use. I always go back to my old ways."

To deal with this situation, recognize that failure is not the end of the world, that it's actually okay to fail if you've genuinely tried to change. But it's also important to learn from past failures to assess what does and doesn't work for you.

To shore up the courage to tackle diet change, take a hard look at yourself and ask, "What did I do in the past that didn't work?" and "What can I do differently in the future?"

Doing this exercise will help you take responsibility for your previous failures, and help you map out a strategy to avoid those pitfalls again. Listing your past successes also helps bolster your confidence.

It's also important to reward yourself with special treats when you're first getting started. For example, at the end of a week in which you incorporated one or two small healthful changes into your diet, treat yourself to a massage or a movie. It's your game, so you decide the prize.

ers' market, although high-quality produce is also available at the sizeable hypermarkets that can be found on the outskirts of nearly every major city, such as Paris, Lyon, and Marseilles.

Healthy food shopping also includes eyeing the expiration date. It's common to check eggs before buying them, for example, to see if they're cracked. The French, on the other hand, are apt to look for the date the eggs were laid, which, in France, is individually stamped on each egg in the carton. This attention to detail is often passed down from parents to children. An American woman in the south of France relates: "A friend's son, who was eleven at the time, came to visit and asked for Coke, which is quite a treat for a French child to have. I told him I had some in the storage room. When he came back without it, I asked him if he found it, and he said, 'Oh, it was out of date.' In other words, if it's past the expiration date, it's not consumable, no matter how much you really want it."

Does anyone other than the French have time for all of this food fussiness? Perhaps, but you probably don't. Still, healthy eating is more than taking in the right mix of nutrients. Like petting your cat or dog or turning off your beeper, there's something to be said for sustaining well-being and maximizing your sense of satisfaction by occasionally whipping up a home-cooked meal that's too good to rush through.

> Also, recognize how the changes you're initiating are making you feel. Do you feel healthier, more energized? These are the real markers of success. Pay attention to them.
>
> And remember, change your diet gradually. Taking one easy step at a time is the best way to make new diet habits a lifelong reality.

Food for Thought

Good news: It's getting faster and easier to cook from scratch. These days, recipe developers are using simple terms instead of run-for-the-dictionary cooking jargon. For example, French-inspired instructions such as "dredge" and "truss" are replaced with the more literal commands "coat with flour" and "close open cavity with string."

French Dietary Guidelines

Like the USDA dietary guidelines, the French Dietary Guidelines, called Seven Tips for Health, emphasize choosing a varied low-fat diet that's moderate in alcohol and contains plenty of fruits and vegetables. Note that although dieting is downplayed in the French culture, keeping tabs on one's weight is a national concern, as stated in dietary guideline #7.

1 Have regular meals.
2 Eat a variety of foods.
3 Fruit and vegetables should be a priority in the diet.
4 Do not abuse fats.
5 If you drink alcohol, drink with moderation.
6 Be active.
7 Weigh yourself every month. (Source: European Food Information Council.)

JAPAN

East Embracing West Beautifully and Healthfully

How beautiful—
Red peppers
After the
autumn gale.

—Yosa Buson

How cold—
Freshly washed
White leeks.

—Matsuo Bashō

For centuries, the Japanese diet has been loaded with carbohydrates, low in protein, and practically devoid of fat. But now, U.S.-style fast food has come to the Land of the Rising Sun, and you can't help but notice that the Japanese diet is, to some extent, on the fat track. Visit Japan today, and you'll see Makadonaldos (McDonald's), for example, dotting the streets in Tokyo and on Okinawa. Turn on Japanese TV, and you'll find cooking programs such as "Dinner in 20 Minutes" (which is an unusually tight time in traditional Japanese cooking).

"Lifestyles have been changing as a consequence of social trends such as changing family structures, increasing employment of women, and interest in spending leisure time more meaningfully," states the *Annual Report on Health and Welfare* from Japan's Ministry of Health and Welfare. As a result, more Japanese are eating out and relying on frozen and processed foods as well as prepared delicacies.

Quick to adopt food trends, "the Japanese love to copy and imitate other cultures," says Lucy Seligman, the owner of Lucy's Kitchen, a Japanese cooking school in Richmond, California. "Then, they refine a food trend into a style or taste that fits the Japanese palate." The present Japanese diet is truly an amalgamation of East and West (and not the best of the West either), especially in Japan's cities where, for example, breakfasts of fried eggs, thick white bread, undercooked bacon, and coffee are not uncommon. But not to worry. The traditional Japanese diet—the one that has the healthy reputation—lives on.

Why the Traditional Japanese Diet Is Worth Importing

As in America, cost and convenience rate high among the Japanese as the basis of their food selections. But surveys show that "ritual and habit" also factor in to the equation. Traditional Japanese cooking still captivates the culinary scene, and perhaps as a result, the Japanese diet remains comparatively lean. In 1960, a meager 10 percent of their calories came from fat. Today, that figure is up to 26 percent. But it still beats the North American diet—we get 34 percent of our calories from fat. And consider this: According to the American Heart Association, the Japanese report death rates from heart disease that are roughly half that of the United States. In fact, according to the AHA's data bank of international statistics, the cardiovascular death rates in Japan rank lowest among thirty-six selected countries. Japan also reports one of the lowest incidences of breast cancer in the world. Type 2 diabetes is also less frequent there than in Western countries, and death rates from breast, prostate, and uterine cancers are stellar by comparison. Certain Japanese cities also report the lowest incidences worldwide of lip, mouth, and throat cancers and Hodgkin's disease (cancer of the lymphatic system). And finally, the Japanese boast the world's highest life expectancy—age seventy-six for men and eighty-two for women.

How Do the Japanese Do It?

Research suggests that the secret to their superior health profile and longevity is not entirely in the genes. Numerous studies have shown, for example, that when the Japanese migrate west and assimilate their eating habits as well as other aspects of their lifestyles accordingly, their disease risk begins to gradually mirror that of their adopted country. And of course, the traditional Japanese diet isn't perfect. Although their death rate from stomach cancer has been declining over the past twenty years, it is still more than seven times that of the United States. The world's highest incidence of stomach cancer is reported in Yamagata, Japan, a thriving northern industrial city. This exceptionally high incidence countrywide is the result of the high amounts of sodium consumed in a diet laden with large quantities of smoked, grilled, salted, and pickled foods. These foods may also contain toxic chemicals such as heterocyclic amines that stimulate the production of pro-inflammatory free radicals, substances that are linked to an increased risk of cancers of the colon, breast, pancreas, bladder, and stomach.

For the most part, however, the Japanese are still on a healthier track, so much so that except in the case of stomach cancer, their positive health factors overcome their negative ones. Based on their health profile and their national longevity, the Japanese are clearly doing something right and have been for centuries. How can you benefit? The following are key diet and health secrets from the culture of the people who live longer than any others.

Japan at a Glance

The diet is one of the world's lowest in fat

- The Japanese get 26 percent of their calories from fat—about 8 percent less fat than found in the typical North American diet. An estimated 65 percent of their calories come from carbohydrates such as rice. It will be interesting to see if the Japanese maintain their health advantages if the proportion of fat calories in their diet continues to rise. Perhaps in the not-too-distant future, the Japanese government will need to initiate an "Eat the Traditional Japanese Diet" public health campaign.

Fish is a mainstay in the traditional Japanese diet

- The omega-3 fatty acids contained in fish likely help reduce the risk of heart disease as well as improve brain function.

Soy foods also play a major role

- Soybeans contain isoflavones—weak, estrogenlike substances that have been associated with many health benefits, including inhibiting the growth of breast and prostate cancer cells, two types of cancer the Japanese have much lower rates of than do North Americans.

Style counts—but not over substance

- The Japanese care about appearances. Even the humblest foods such as rice don't come to the table disheveled. Historically, this focus on food presentation served the purpose of transforming a low-fat, low-calorie cuisine into one that was appetizing and thus more satisfying.

The Japanese report low rates of major chronic diseases

- The Japanese report death rates from heart disease that are half that of the United States, as well as one of the lowest incidences of breast cancer in the world. Type 2 (non-insulin-dependent) diabetes is also less frequent in Japan than in Western countries, and death rates from breast, prostate, and uterine cancers are comparatively low.

The Japanese live longest

- They boast the world's highest life expectancy—age seventy-six for men and eighty-two for women.

GLOBAL EATING SECRET #20

Make Low-Cal, Low-Fat Foods Look Good

During the sixth century, when the Japanese government introduced Buddhism, consuming the flesh of "four-leggeds"—the flesh of animals—was ruled forbidden, as was the flesh of fowl. This culinary tradition lasted until the final third of the nineteenth century, until the end of Japan's national seclusion. That period had begun in 1625 when Japan closed its doors almost completely to overseas contacts of any kind and thus became the only non-European country never to be colonized. By eliminating an entire food group, the Japanese diet moved into a healthy arena; what was left to eat—soup, rice, pickles, soy foods, fresh vegetables, and the bounty from the sea—was virtually fat free.

Each of these foods, especially steamed white short-grain rice, continues to be a staple in the Japanese diet. The Japanese get roughly 65 percent of their total daily calories from carbohydrates, mostly from white rice, called *gohan*, which also means "meal." Granted, the Japanese also love their noodles. *Udon* (wheat-based noodles) or *soba* (noodles made from buckwheat flour) regularly pinch-hit for rice, as do barley, millet, or sweet potatoes, albeit less frequently than noodles.

Since the present majority of residents of the Japanese archipelago came from the Chinese mainland several millennia ago, it's no wonder that rice is at the center of their cuisine. "You literally can't talk about eating in Japan unless you talk about rice. When someone doesn't have rice at a meal, they make a point of noting its absence," says Elizabeth Andoh, an American who runs A Taste of Culture, a Tokyo cooking school that caters to business people who've been transferred to Japan and find themselves overwhelmed in the most foreign of territories—a Japanese food market. (If there's a Japanese market in your neighborhood, visit it one day to get an idea of what this feels like. The market will no doubt be filled with an assortment of edibles that you won't be able to identify, unless you're fluent in the language.)

Food as Art

To make fish, rice, soy, and vegetables more appetizing, the Japanese have traditionally prepared meals to "be eaten with the eyes." Food isn't served as much as it's displayed. The visual aesthetics of food presentation is a central element of the culture. Prized in Japan is simple food that's fashioned with attention to detail, color, form, and balance, with serving dishes functioning much like a painter's canvas. The Japanese believe, for example, that a humble portion of white rice or a morsel of tofu looks much more appealing when presented in a black lacquer bowl; that vegetables can make your mouth water when artfully arranged on just the right oblong ceramic or bamboo "plate" and garnished with leaves or flowers from the garden. If you haven't noticed this already, do so the next time you're at a Japanese restaurant. Almost without exception, whatever you order is bound to be presented in a meticulous and symmetrical mosaic of shapes, colors, textures, and tastes.

Compared to Western table settings in which, very often, an entire meal is served on one plate, the traditional Japanese table is scattered with various small dishes, each for a specific food, each of different design, yet all harmoniously coordinated. Why the fuss? "Presentation is very important because it stimulates the appetite," says Kiyoko Konishi, owner of Konishi Japanese Cooking, a Tokyo cooking school she has been running for thirty years. "Good presentation means we use lots of different ingredients, so the meal is well balanced. Different kinds of vegetables as side dishes make it look much prettier."

For many North Americans, a porterhouse steak dripping in its own juice needs little fanfare. But if you're trying to cut down on these kinds of hefty foods for the sake of your heart and your general health, take a hint from the Japanese. To make lower-calorie, lower-fat foods more tempting and satisfying, don't nosh out of the takeout carton or glom food onto your plate as if it were the consolation prize. Dress it up before you dig in. Make it look good.

Food for Thought

In Chinese and Japanese diets, where rice has customarily been considered the body's principal fuel, salty foods like pickles served (as they still do) the purpose of accenting the blandness of rice to coax partakers to eat more of this life-sustaining grain.

Food for Thought

In Japan as in America, it is mainly women who are responsible for what the family eats. Currently, more women are working outside the home than have in the past, but many Japanese mothers still spend hours each morning assembling the healthy obento, a traditional box lunch, for their school-age children, as they have for decades. The obento features white rice and an assortment of tiny seasonal helpings of meat, fish, vegetables, egg, and perhaps a tiny pickled plum (umeboshi), all neatly arranged in a small lacquered rectangular box.

Eat More Fish Meals

A Note from Dr. Jonas
GRADUAL CHANGE LEADS TO PERMANENT CHANGES

This is one of my favorite sayings about any personal health-promoting behavior change—whether it's becoming a healthy eater, a regular exerciser, or someone who manages stress well. The person who changes by taking a series of small steps and building on each one slowly, gradually, and carefully, is much more likely to achieve success in terms of permanent change than is the person who tries to go all out right away.

Let's say you're now eating a rather high-fat diet, especially a high-fat dinner, replete with red meat, a baked potato with lots of butter or sour cream, and a delicious but high-fat salad dressing such as blue cheese, five times a week. Let's also say that you're willing to let this book inspire you to change your ways. If so, next week, don't try to immediately replace all of those dinners with healthy ones drawn from the suggested recipes and menus, starting on page 117. Instead, go from five to four fat-rich suppers for a week or two, then to three for another two weeks, substituting healthy meals for them.

Even better, start with smaller changes. For example, for the first week, just replace the regular sour cream on your baked potato with a low-fat brand. The next week, also switch to low-fat blue cheese dressing, and so on. Before you know it, you'll only be eating one or two high-fat items at dinner (which is okay), and you won't even know how you got there.

On average, the Japanese annually consume more than 45 pounds of fish per capita—about three times more per capita than North Americans. As an island nation, Japan has been mining its seas for centuries. "How to master the use of seafood is a very important matter here," says Kiyoko Konishi, the Tokyo cooking school proprietor.

Fish is rich in protein and is generally lower in fat than beef or chicken. It can also provide good doses of iron and zinc. If the fish contains bones that are ground to be served with the flesh (such as canned salmon), you can count on getting calcium and phosphorus, too, which can help fight osteoporosis. Many Japanese eat fish at least once a day. That's asking a lot of a Westerner, but here's why you should consider eating fish at least once or twice a week.

Fish Is Heart Healthy

Many types of fish contain a small amount of a special group of essential omega-3 fatty acids ("essential" because your body can't make them on its own, yet needs them to function). You can only get omega-3s from your diet. Studies on omega-3s suggest that this "good" fat may help reduce the risk of heart disease (unlike the artery-clogging saturated fat found in animal foods such as red meat and butter). That the average Japanese consumes omega-3s regularly is perhaps one of the reasons why the rates of heart disease in Japan are much lower than in North America. One U.S. study that followed 1,800 men from the Chicago area for thirty years, found that those who ate at least 8 ounces of omega-3–rich fish weekly had a 40 percent lower risk of fatal heart attack than those who ate no fish at all.

And omega-3s are polyunsaturated fatty acids. Compared to the saturated fat hidden in meat, omega-3s make blood clotting more difficult and change how the walls of your blood vessels interact with different cells in the blood. By consuming a diet rich in omega-3s, you prime your arteries to relax, therefore making them less likely to clog and impair the blood circulation of your heart. Omega-3s may also change the chemistry in the heart that affects heartbeat, the flow of blood, and the chemical reactions in blood vessels.

Omega-3s reside mainly in fatty fish such as salmon, bluefish, sardines, herring, and mackerel, all of which are prevalent in the Japanese diet. Lower-fat choices include cod, tuna, and haddock, all of which are rich sources of omega-3s. Shellfish, such as clams, shrimp, and lobster, however, are not a significant omega-3 source.

Fish Is Brain Food

Besides being heart healthy, the omega-3s found in fish may also provide your brain with more wattage to help you think more clearly. After all, fat is a major component of brain tissue, and omega-3s continually flood the brain's synaptic membranes (connections from one brain cell to the next) that form its circuitry. The brain's synaptic membranes contain essential fatty acids you can only get from food. Moreover, recent studies show that consuming omega-3 fatty acids may reduce the symptoms of a variety of psychiatric illnesses, including schizophrenia, bipolar disorder, and depression. For unborn babies and newborns, DHA (a type of omega-3 fatty acid that is transferred through the placenta and breast milk) is also believed to be important for eye and brain development.

Your Mission: Get Savvy at the Seafood Counter

From snapper to sole, tilapia to tilefish, the number of options at your supermarket's fish counter can be confusing. To alleviate any trepidation you may have, and to help you get into the habit of eating fish regularly, get acquainted with someone behind the counter and ask him or her for a recommendation. Explain what you like in the way of flavor and texture, and ask for a suggestion and what kinds of fish are in season. The price can usually give you a

Food for Thought

A traditional Japanese breakfast (asa gohan) *often includes fish. To cut cooking time, the Japanese typically prepare a breakfast fish that's been partially dried, which cooks in five minutes. Lunch* (hiru gohan) *is lighter and faster, and may not include any sea creatures aside from dashi (miso-fish broth). But you can count on fish (along with soup, rice, and pickles) to make an appearance again at dinner* (ban gohan), *which tends to take place at 8:30 or 9:00 P.M., at the end of a very long workday.*

> **A Note from Dr. Jonas**
> ## A WARNING TO MOTHERS
> ## AND MOTHERS-TO-BE
>
> If you're pregnant or breast-feeding, the U.S. National Academy of Sciences recommends limiting your consumption of shark, swordfish, and fresh tuna to once a month. The academy also suggests avoiding all raw and undercooked fish and shellfish, particularly clams, mussels, and oysters. These seafoods may contain pollutants and chemical contaminants that could be harmful to your baby.

hint: In-season fish are often the best deal at the fish counter.

If your supermarket doesn't offer fresh fish, don't worry. Frozen fish is just as nutritious and rich in omega-3s as its fresh counterpart. In fact, depending on the part of the country where you live, much of the "fresh" fish at your market's fish counter may have already been frozen, then thawed. (Fish that has been frozen should be labeled "previously frozen.")

A trick to trying fish: Think about how you'd like chicken prepared and what flavors you like, such as teriyaki chicken, then transfer those tastes to seafood. In general, fish will take on the flavor you add to it.

Food for Thought

In 1971, McDonald's first opened its doors on the opulent Ginza, the world-famous shopping area in Tokyo that was home to the city's first department stores. Since then, more than 2,400 Makadonaldos have hoisted their golden arches in Japan, serving millions of daily orders of U.S. and regional specialties, such as the Teriyaki McBurger—a sausage patty on a bun with teriyaki sauce, a product that was created specifically to meet local demand.

Tips for Cooking Fish

To cook fish, stick to no-fail "moist" techniques, such as poaching, steaming, microwaving, and baking. As the Japanese have learned from centuries of fish finessing, with moist-preparation methods, the fish never dries out, even if you cook it longer than necessary. As a general rule, cook fish for ten minutes for every inch of thickness in a 400°F to a 450°F oven. Add five minutes to the total cooking time for fish wrapped in foil or covered in sauce. Double the cooking time for unthawed fish. You'll know it's done when it flakes with a fork.

Seafood Safety

Trust your nose to know whether fish is safe to eat. The fish you buy should smell pleasant and not have a strong fishy smell. Here are some other clues that the fish you're considering is safe to eat and of high quality.

- The seafood counter is clean, and the fish is packed well in ice.
- The edges of the fish aren't dry.
- For finfish, such as swordfish and tuna, the flesh is moist, clear, and firm to the touch.

- If frozen or fresh fish is wrapped, it should be wrapped tightly. The shells of the shellfish aren't broken.
- If you're buying frozen fish, it's frozen hard, not half-thawed.

Once you get your catch home, put it in the freezer immediately if it's frozen and you don't plan to eat it that night. If it's fresh and you plan to eat it soon, wash it under cold running water, pat dry, wrap in plastic wrap, and place in an airtight container. (For whole fish, also fill the body cavity with ice.) Store fresh fish in the coldest part of your refrigerator (32°F to 40°F). This is usually in the meat drawer or in the middle of the back of the refrigerator. Stored correctly, both fresh fish and fish that has been frozen and then thawed will keep for up to four days.

--------- G L O B A L   E A T I N G   S E C R E T   # 22 ---------

Give Soy Foods a Try

An excellent source of vegetable protein, soy is a Japanese tradition. One of the core components of the Japanese diet, soy is believed to have originated in the Muromachi period (1333–1568), when tofu, a custardlike white substance made from curdled soy milk and natto (fermented soybeans) made its debut on the food scene. According to estimates, the Japanese average 7 to 10 grams of soy protein each day. For breakfast, you can expect to sip broth thickened with miso, which is a fermented soybean paste that's a basic flavoring in Japanese cooking. At lunch and dinner, you might find *agedashi* tofu—delicately fried bean curd in tempura sauce; *hiya yako*—cold soft tofu served with fresh grated ginger and flakes of dried bonito (tuna); *sukiyaki*—a stew that regardless of what other components it might contain, always features tofu; or *yosenabe* ("a gathering of everything"), which may include tofu, seafood,

Food for Thought

Dashi, *a basic stock made from giant kelp (seaweed) and dried bonito (tuna) flakes, is often referred to as the backbone of Japanese cuisine. Commonly flavored with soy sauce, sake, and mirin (sweet sake for cooking), it's the medium for nearly all Japanese vegetable dishes, clear soups, and simmered dishes. In fact, it's the basis of the miso soup you order at any Japanese restaurant.*

A Note from Dr. Jonas
SAFER SUSHI

Centuries ago, the Japanese invented sushi (bite-size pieces of raw fish seasoned with wasabi [Japanese horseradish] and wrapped around or layered with boiled rice flavored with vinegar) and sashimi (individual pieces of raw fish served with condiments such as daikon radish, ginger root, wasabi, and soy sauce). In North America, the word "sushi" is generically applied to both types of fish. Sushi has become a national favorite both in Japan and abroad. In the United States, individual sushi meals are now sold in many urban supermarkets and delis, as well as at sushi bars and restaurants. It's a taste treat that inspires cravings, and in Japan, sushi occupies the position of culinary royalty to be prepared by the masters wielding a knife as sharp as a samurai sword, rather than at home. But no matter where you get your sushi, beware. Some raw or undercooked finfish such as tuna and salmon may contain *Anisakis simplex* (anisakid nematodes) and related wormy parasites or bacteria that can cause illness.

Fortunately, according to the Centers for Disease Control, "bad bugs" from fish are rare in the United States. Fewer than ten cases of parasitic infections from raw or undercooked seafood are diagnosed in the United States annually. (The Japanese, however, aren't so lucky; they have the highest number of reported cases due to the large volume of raw fish consumed there.) Nevertheless, the U.S. Food and Drug Administration (FDA) recommends that all fish and shellfish intended for raw or semiraw use be blast frozen at −31°F or below for fifteen hours, or frozen at −4°F or below for seven days.

If you're pregnant or your immune system is weakened, it's a very good idea to play it safe by ordering only maki, sushi rolls made with vegetables, cooked fish, or fish roe that are wrapped in thin sheets of nori (seaweed). Look for these: Kappa-Maki (cucumber roll), California Roll (avocado and cooked crab), Kampyo-Maki (sushi made with gourd strips), Natto-Maki (sushi made with fermented soybeans), Futo-Maki (sushi made with vegetables and cooked eggs), Tako (sushi made with cooked octopus), Ika (sushi made with cooked squid), Anago (sushi made with cooked eel), and Ebi (sushi made with cooked shrimp). If you just have to have sushi and sashimi and you're willing to risk it, consider eating only items that have been prepared at reputable restaurants. At the sushi bar, you may also want to ask if the fish has been frozen and for how long.

meat, vegetables, and noodles swimming in broth.

"Soy is also commonly used in salad dressings, as a thickening for soups, as a dip for crudité, as a seasoning for meatloaf," says Elizabeth Andoh, the Japanese cooking school instructor. In Japan, you won't find the tofu hot dogs, hamburgers, ready-made salad dressings, tofu salads, and soy dips you often see in North American supermarkets and health food stores. The Japanese are known to use soy in its basic forms—tofu, miso, and natto—and to prepare it hundreds of ways.

During that long stretch when Buddhism, which forbade meat consumption, was the dominant religion in Japan, tofu was an all-important source of protein. "Miso and soy played the dual role of adding meatlike flavor to the Japanese diet," says William Shurtleff, director of the Soy Foods Center and author of *The Book of Tofu*, who lived in Japan for six years. Today, even with the influx of the Western-style diet, the Japanese, on average, still eat only about 3 ounces of meat daily, which is a serving about the size of a floppy disk. One of the reasons is that meat in Japan is an expensive commodity.

The Health Benefits of Soy Foods

Because they're made from plants, soy foods have no cholesterol and may reduce the level of LDL (the "bad" cholesterol) in the blood, which makes them particularly heart healthy. Another major plus: Many soy foods—tofu, tempeh (fermented bean curd), soy milk, tofu hot dogs and burgers, miso (fermented soybeans, often used for flavoring in Japanese cooking), soy cheese, and soy flour—are cancer fighters, particularly against breast and prostate cancers, of which the Japanese have much lower rates than do North Americans. (One caveat: Hold the soy sauce, which doesn't help combat cancer because it doesn't contain isoflavones.)

Soy foods house powerful phytochemicals called isoflavones, estrogen-like substances made by plants. Isoflavones can act as a form of the estrogen needed by menopausal women. By mimicking estrogen, isoflavones may also help coronary arteries become more elastic, enabling them to dilate promptly on cue and thus reducing the risk of heart attack.

Isoflavones may also hinder the growth of prostate cancer cells and inhibit blood vessel formation around tumors as well as block tumor-causing enzymes. Moreover, isoflavones have been associated with a reduced risk of osteoporosis (which is linked to inadequate estrogen levels in the blood). Asian women tend to eat less animal protein than do North American women, another factor that may account for the incidence of osteoporosis in Asia being lower than in the United States. In general, the more animal protein you consume, the more protein you excrete, which may compromise bone health, especially postmenopause. Asian and Caucasian women share many of the risk factors for osteoporosis, including a thin, small-boned frame and a diet low in calcium. For Asian women, the average calcium intake, which is essential for building and maintaining a healthy skeleton, is estimated to be about half that of Western populations. Yet, studies show that Asian women have lower hip fracture rates than Caucasian women. In studies involving rats whose ovaries are removed, soy protein prevents the subsequent bone loss.

It's well documented that when you reduce your consumption of animal foods and substitute them with plant-based foods such as soy, you're likely to reduce the serum cholesterol and triglyceride levels in your blood and improve your overall heart disease–risk profile. But scientific investigations into the role of soy and isoflavones in protecting health are still in the preliminary stages. All the cancer-preventive benefits of soy, for example, have yet to be discovered. But in the meantime, it's safe to say that men and women (both pre- and postmenopausal) stand to benefit from increasing their intake of this bean-based food.

Soy Foods 101: Getting Started

As mentioned earlier, besides containing isoflavones, soy foods are a good source of protein, calcium, and complex carbohydrates. Regarding flavor, a concern many of us share, tofu in particular has little of its own, but it easily

Food for Thought

Nori, the seaweed wrapper surrounding the rolled version of sushi (maki), is also a decent source of omega-3 fatty acids. In fact, fish get their omega-3 fatty acids from the seaweed in their diet.

Food for Thought

An ume, a Japanese plum that's salt-cured and sun-dried for several days to yield a wrinkled pink umeboshi, is often served at breakfast in Japan, smack in the middle of one's rice bowl. Since ancient times, the umeboshi is believed to have medicinal properties. In fact, it contains generous amounts of vitamin C (and a dose of MSG). On New Year's Day, one umeboshi is often placed in the morning's first tea to assure good health all year long.

A Note from Dr. Jonas
SOY AND HOT FLASHES

If you've been paying attention to the media reports of the dozens of research studies on benefits of soy that are popping up in medical journals, you know about the promising results that soy has shown in connection with hot flashes, which many women experience during menopause. During a hot flash, which is triggered by a decrease in estrogen levels and usually lasts from thirty seconds to five minutes several times a day or at night, the skin on the head and neck becomes red and hot, and profuse sweating can occur. It has been reported that, compared to North American women, fewer Asian women complain of these menopausal symptoms. Research suggests, however, that menopausal problems are indeed a common topic of conversation among Japanese women at that stage of life.

In any event, in one study conducted at the Menopause and Osteoporosis Center at the University of Ferrara in Italy, 51 of 104 patients ranging in age from forty-eight to sixty-one consumed 60 grams of isolated soy protein daily for twelve weeks. The remaining 53 consumed a placebo. The study concluded that soy protein was significantly superior to the placebo. By the end of the twelfth week, patients taking soy had a 45 percent reduction in their daily hot flashes versus a 30 percent reduction obtained in the placebo group.

Hundreds of studies cite similar findings and support the theory that phytoestrogens such as the isoflavones in soy protein may reduce menopausal symptoms and offer protective effects on bones and the cardiovascular system. According to the National Menopause Society, many short-term menopause-related effects may be eased by eating daily a portion of soy-containing foods (soy milk,

absorbs the flavors of marinades and seasonings. This makes it perfect for a variety of dishes. The basic types of tofu—soft (or silken), firm, and extra firm—are available in the produce aisle of most supermarkets. Although the jury is still out on whether soy foods can help reduce your risk of heart disease, osteoporosis, and cancer, they're a smart substitute for meat on occasion. Here are some easy ways to add soy to your diet:

- Substitute soft tofu for cream cheese in recipes.
- Use firm tofu in place of eggs in egg salad.
- Add firm tofu cubes to a vegetable stir-fry.
- Spread miso (typically available at health food stores and Japanese markets) on grilled eggplant.
- If you're lactose intolerant or otherwise don't drink milk, consider soy milk, which is lactose free. For best protection against osteoporosis, seek brands that have been fortified with calcium (check the label).

Japanese Dietary Guidelines

To stay healthy in Japan, you're on the right track if you:

1 Obtain well-balanced nutrition with a variety of foods; eat thirty foodstuffs a day.
2 Take energy corresponding to daily activity. (Match your calorie intake with your activity level.)
3 Consider the amount and quality of the fats and oils you eat; avoid eating too much fat; eat more vegetable oils than animal fat.

4 Avoid too much salt, not more than 10 grams a day.

5 Sit down and eat together and talk; treasure family time and home cooking. Happy eating makes for happy family life.

Besides basic nutrition recommendations, as you can see the Dietary Guidelines for the Japanese, developed by the Japanese government, stress eating together as a family, which is considered an occasion for happiness and a way to promote cultural tradition. However, a long workday—as late as 10:30 P.M. each night—is the custom in Japan, which often precludes families from eating the main meal together. This luxury is commonly reserved for Sundays, when everyone has more time at home.

---

soybeans, tofu). But how much soy to eat to achieve the benefits has not been scientifically documented. A 3-ounce portion of tofu—equal to one serving of meat, is a safe place to start. And keep in mind that even if soy foods don't technically help ease menopause symptoms, you shouldn't discount the placebo effect. Eating soy and merely thinking it will help ease your menopausal symptoms may be enough to do the trick.

Diabetes—Lessons from Japanese Americans

Undiagnosed and untreated, diabetes can threaten your life. According to the National Institute of Diabetes and Digestive and Kidney Diseases, approximately 15 million Americans have diabetes, half of whom have yet to be medically diagnosed, which is more than three times the number in 1958. Nine out of ten cases are Type 2, the condition in which (1) your pancreas doesn't make enough insulin, the hormone that helps convert the food you eat to energy, or (2) your cells resist the insulin your pancreas makes. (Type 1 is an inherited condition that typically starts in childhood in which your pancreas stops making insulin entirely.) If not diagnosed early and managed properly, Type 2 diabetes can kill you just as swiftly and silently as heart disease can. It can also lead to blindness, nerve damage, limb amputations, and kidney failure.

Compared to North Americans, the Japanese report a much lower incidence of diabetes. However, it's steadily on the rise, especially among Japanese schoolchildren, who are consuming four times more animal fat now than they did in 1975.

Moreover, when the Japanese settle in the United States, for example, and their diet Westernizes, the prevalence of Type 2 diabetes among them increases dramatically. That rise is possibly due to a diet that includes higher amounts of animal protein and fat, which can lead to weight gain. Among other things, excess weight makes your pancreas work harder to produce extra

A Note from Dr. Jonas
WELLNESS IS A JOURNEY

To become a healthy eater, consider yourself on a lifelong journey, one in which there's no final destination. In fact, there can never be one because there are always new healthy foods, cuisines, and habits to explore and enjoy. All told, wellness through a healthy diet is a way of life, not an endpoint. This book hopes to show you how to make healthy eating a continuous adventure, not a temporary test of your endurance and willpower.

insulin. If you also have a genetic predisposition for diabetes, your pancreas eventually won't be able to keep up, insulin levels will start to fall, and diabetes will result in due time. One of the most easily detectable early signs of Type 2 diabetes is a rising blood sugar level.

To minimize, delay, or possibly even prevent the onset of Type 2 diabetes and its complications, *don't* do as the Japanese do who migrate here. Make efforts to guard against weight gain, especially if you're over forty. If you already have Type I or Type 2 diabetes and you're overweight, shedding as little as 10 to 15 pounds can help make your cells more receptive to insulin to prevent some diabetes complications.

--- GLOBAL EATING SECRET #23 ---

Celebrate the Seasons with Food

Food for Thought

Though nearly dairy-free, the Japanese diet relies heavily on dried seaweed such as hijiki *and* wakame *(wah-ka-may) for calcium. By U.S. standards, a few tablespoons of reconstituted* hijiki, *for example, provides 15 percent of the recommended dietary allowance for calcium.* Hijiki *and* wakame *can be found in Asian markets. To prepare, soak in cold water for thirty minutes. Drain and add to soups, salads, meat and vegetable dishes for a calcium boost.*

Forget about hot-house strawberries in January or cantaloupe in April. While most produce available in North American supermarkets is always in good supply, it's quintessentially Japanese to plan meals with the seasons in mind. "Each season has its own special gifts from nature," says Kiyoko Konishi. Depending on the time of the year, specific fruits and vegetables—even seafood—in Japan are highlighted and mined for their culinary possibilities. A true Japanese chef is the one who can take a single, humble, in-season vegetable, such as a lowly sweet potato, and make a banquet of twelve delicious courses.

Japanese tastes are in harmony with nature. Summer is the time for grilled eel, octopus, abalone, and plenty of fresh fruits and vegetables. Late autumn is the occasion for *matsutake*, a highly-prized mushroom coveted for its distinctive fragrance and taste, and for preserving the summer's vegetable bounty. Besides being the best buy, foods in season usually offer more taste and nutrients—including vitamins, minerals, and natural disease-fighting phytochemicals (plant chemicals that don't have nutritional value but have beneficial biological activity in the body), which may reduce the risk of cancer and other diseases. In-season produce is often the brightest and most deeply colored, a sign of peak nutrient content.

How Sumo Wrestlers Get So Fat

Sumo wrestling is a 2,000-year-old sport in which two 400-plus-pound wrestlers lunge at each other very briefly, attempting to force each other out of a circle 15 feet in diameter, or to cause an opponent's body part (other than the soles of his feet) to touch the ground. Roundly contrasting the typical Japanese, sumo wrestlers get their size from a regime of muscle-building exercises and two daily gargantuan meals of *chanko-nabe*, a kitchen-sink stew brimming with meat (post-Buddhism), fish, and vegetables, as well as anything else that may be on hand. To fortify this daily gluttony, sumo wrestlers also consume thousands of calories via endless bowls of rice, sushi (as many as seventy pieces in one sitting), and numerous bottles of beer—and cap it all off with a lengthy postlunch nap.

SCANDINAVIA
The Benefits of Dairy and Grains

*If there's no bread in the
house, there's nothing to eat.*

—Anonymous, popular
Finnish sentiment

In the past, to consume the Scandinavian diet was to exist on a smorgasbord of hot boiled potatoes; meat; smoked reindeer; smoked salmon, whitefish, or Baltic herring; rich chunky beef stews such as the hearty Norwegian *oksegryte*; homemade cheeses; milk that could pass for cream; and bread or *flatbrod* (thin, crackerlike bread) heaped with cheese or ample smears of butter. Why such a rich diet? For much of the year, the outside temperature registers below zero. The extra calories were needed to fend off that arctic chill. And besides, a bounty of fruits and vegetables in this frozen hinterland simply wasn't available.

Not surprisingly, the traditional diet of Scandinavia was nothing the health-minded eater would care to emulate. Its high-fat content was likely related to the off-the-chart rates of cardiovascular disease and cancer incidence and mortality reported for decades in the land of the midnight sun.

Fortunately, however, the Scandinavian diet is changing and so is the health profile of Sweden, Denmark, Norway, and Finland (which isn't ethnically part of Scandinavia, but is very much so in spirit). For example, the hearts of the Finnish people are getting healthier in major part because of a national public health program to achieve that result. In the past, their rates of heart disease death hovered among the world's highest, especially in the eastern part of the country. Between 1972 and 1992, however, heart disease mortality plummeted 55 percent among men and nearly 70 percent among women.

Similarly, in Norway, deaths from heart disease have also declined sharply since the late 1970s—by 40 percent in the forty- to forty-nine-year-

Food for Thought

When Finnish heart disease rates peaked in the mid–twentieth century, so did their consumption of "boiled" coffee, the conventional full-bodied brew of Finland. After much research, epidemiologists determined that two compounds in the Finnish coffee—cafestol and kahweol—were elevating total serum cholesterol levels and LDL (bad) cholesterol. But it wasn't the beans they were using or the water that led to the high levels of these harmful chemicals in their coffee. It was the way they made it. The Finnish recipe for a heart attack: Place coffee grounds directly in boiling water. Boil for a little while and set aside. Boil grounds in the same water two more times. Strain and serve.

The Finns, a conventionally frugal people, were attempting to boil as much flavor as they could out of the ground coffee beans, which are an expensive commodity. But researchers found that when coffee is prepared this way, sans a coffee filter, and consumed several times a day for

old age group. More modest success in curbing heart disease holds true for Sweden. Nevertheless, their life expectancy continues to rise and is now on a par with the United States.

Moreover, according to World Health Organization statistics, the incidences of breast, prostate, lung, and colorectal cancers—four major killers in the United States—remain significantly less of a threat in this corner of the world. With these statistics in mind, you have to ask, What's their secret?

Nordic Nuances

Like many Americans, the Swedes, Finns, Norwegians, and Danes are modernizing their eating habits to reduce their risk of diet-related diseases. Thanks to years of aggressive governmental public health campaigns, they're tweaking their diet in ways that are perhaps instructive for North Americans. This chapter fills you in on these improvements as well as the healthy traditions they're hanging on to that are worth importing into your diet.

The Nordic Countries at a Glance

High fiber

- Whole-grain breads and cereals count among the staples of the Scandinavian diet. Consequently, you wouldn't be exaggerating if you called the traditional Nordic diet a fiber fest. As noted earlier, studies show that a high-fiber diet may reduce the risk of heart disease, some forms of cancer, constipation, and other intestinal problems. A high-fiber diet may also prevent and help better manage Type 2 diabetes.

Lower-fat dairy products

- The Scandinavian diet is traditionally high in saturated fat found in plentiful quantities in the dairy products the Nordic people consumed regularly. Now, however, most Nordic markets carry a variety of low-fat and low-salt cheeses, as well as low-fat milk and yogurt. Consequently, their historically high rates of heart disease are dropping in line with the decline in saturated fat intake.

More fruits and vegetables

• Fruits and vegetables don't play a big part in the traditional Scandinavian diet for obvious reasons. However, that's changing as the result of the increased availability of a wide selection of imported produce and the high consumer interest in living a long and healthy life. The governments of Sweden, Denmark, Finland, and Norway are encouraging produce consumption with ambitious "five-a-day" and "six-a-day" public health campaigns, similar to what's going on in the United States and some other countries.

GLOBAL EATING SECRET # 24

Go for Grains

It's an understatement to say that Scandinavians love their whole-grain cereals such as oatmeal, and have an intense affinity for whole-grain bread. In Finland and Norway, especially, breaking bread is an all-day event. "If you speak about Finnish food, you speak about bread," says Jukka Oresto, a food journalist and host of *Bon Appetit*, a national food television show in Finland. "It is very essential in our diet." An integral part of breakfast, lunch, and dinner, bread eating doesn't stop there. It's typically Nordic to follow up with a slice or two in the evening. More so than the potato, which boasts a shorter though prominent role in Nordic culinary history, whole-grain bread, especially rye, is to Scandinavians and the Finns what white rice is to Asians, what french fries are to Americans, what beans and legumes are to the people of the Mediterranean. Although international influences such as the French baguette are making their way to the Nordic region, it's still a common local belief that rye and whole-grain bread is what keeps one healthy, wealthy, and wise.

Fibering Up

As you might suspect, the Scandinavian diet is traditionally loaded with fiber because of their whole-grain habit. Consider these statistics: In Denmark, they typically consume 27 grams of fiber a day (people in the United States average a mere 12 grams a day). A Finn gets two-thirds more fiber each day than a typical North American. Swedish consumers chew their way daily through

days on end, the final product stimulates both total and LDL serum cholesterol production and sends both soaring. Today, the Finns still get their daily caffeine fix; coffee consumption in Finland measures among the world's highest. But cholesterol levels have collectively plunged in Finland thanks to public health campaigns that created a controversy over the boiled coffee–cholesterol connection. Most Finns now make their coffee more conventionally—by pouring hot water over ground coffee in a filter (which filters out both cholesterol-raising compounds). Nonetheless, a passing trend initiated by coffee bars was to brew coffee in a cafetière, otherwise known as a plunger pot or coffee press. It doesn't require a filter. Like Finnish boiled coffee, pressed coffee can raise serum cholesterol levels. Fortunately, this method of coffee brewing got lots of bad press. But if you're still brewing your coffee this way, take a lesson from the Finns and brew your coffee using a paper or gold-meshed filter.

Food for Thought

In Finland, "home baking is popular and bread machines are in constant use," writes Anna-Maija Tanttu, in The Gastronomy of Finland, *for the Ministry for Foreign Affairs. "The range of different types of bread just seems to grow, with new shapes and seasonings being developed all the time."*

Food for Thought

In Norway, the custom throughout the country is to bring your lunch, or "food package," to work because the standard lunch "hour" is twenty to thirty minutes. Thus, it pays to pack foods that you can eat quickly. Invariably, one's food package contains 3 to 5 sizeable slices of rye bread with thin slices of cheese, a custom that has helped the Norwegians earn their reputation as Scandinavia's biggest bread eaters.

roughly 20 grams of fiber. Still, the Swedish government believes Swedes can do better. "The recommendation is to increase fiber to 25 to 30 grams," says Ake Bruce, Ph.D., of the Swedish National Food Administration.

Similarly, the American Heart Association recommends that Americans consume 25 to 30 daily grams of fiber, more than double typical consumption.

Unfortunately, that's not an easily achievable goal. Only 5 percent of the grain foods North Americans now eat are in whole-grain form. The rest are refined grains that have been stripped of much of their fabulous fiber.

The Health Benefits of Whole Grains

Whole-grain foods boost intake of fiber, which is plant material the body can't digest. Fiber is thought to bulk up intestinal waste and then speed it through the digestive tract, cutting down on the body's exposure to cancer-causing agents. For years, epidemiologists believed that eating a high-fiber diet reduced the risk of colon and rectal (colorectal) cancers, the second highest cause of cancer-related death (after lung cancer) in the United States. Now, they're not so sure; a major study published in the *New England Journal of Medicine* discounted the colon cancer theory. The Nurses Health Study, which involved over 88,000 women over a sixteen-year period, found no evidence that a fiber-rich diet, which included whole-grain foods and vegetables, protected against colon cancer. Nevertheless, that observational study was conducted in women only. Many other studies have shown a possibility that there is a link between higher fiber consumption and lower colon cancer risk. Clearly, the link between diet and colon cancer remains controversial, and more research needs to be done to establish or refute the colorectal cancer–fiber theory.

Still, a fiber-rich diet has been shown to be not only protective against cancers of the mouth, throat, stomach, and lungs, but also effective in reducing constipation and other intestinal problems.

Moreover, a diet rich in whole-grain foods has been shown to generally protect against heart attack by lowering LDL (bad) cholesterol and total cholesterol without affecting HDL (good) cholesterol. In fact, a nine-year study conducted by the University of Minnesota, involving more than 30,000 women ages fifty-five to sixty-nine, concluded that those who ate at least three servings of whole grains a day were 30 percent less likely to die of heart attack than those who averaged less than one daily whole-grain serving.

Fiber also plays a part in preventing high blood pressure and Type 2 diabetes. A high-fiber diet may also help you better manage diabetes-related complications.

Whole-grain foods also offer plenty of magnesium (beneficial for fending off osteoporosis and boosting your immune system functioning) and phytochemicals that act as disease-fighting antioxidants, such as heart-healthy vitamin E.

Good News for Weight Watchers

Not only does a high-fiber diet lower your risk of heart disease, cancer, and diabetes, it helps keep you slim. This is one reason why the Swedish government is actively promoting an eat-more-fiber campaign; fiber decreases fat intake. Load up your diet with high-fiber foods, which are often naturally low in fat, and you'll have less room for everything else.

A high-fiber diet can also help you keep your weight in check by helping you absorb fewer fat calories. Case in point: A USDA study concluded that a high-fiber diet helps cut calories by blocking the digestion of some of the fat and protein consumed with it. In the study, participants consumed 18 to 36 grams of fiber a day (one-and-one-half to three times the U.S. national average) and absorbed 130 fewer daily calories. Do the math. That adds up to a deficit of 47,450 calories—the number of calories it would take to produce 13 pounds of body weight—over a year's time. To boost the fiber in their diet, participants generally made simple switches such as eating whole-wheat bread (2 grams of fiber/slice) instead of white bread (<1 gram of fiber/slice) and noshing on apples (3.5 grams of fiber/apple) instead of drinking apple juice (<1 gram of fiber/4 oz. glass).

Are You Getting Enough Fiber?

While eating more fiber is a culinary custom worth importing, there's a catch to trying to do it the Scandinavian way in North America. Traditional

---

A Note from Dr. Jonas
THE HEART-HEALTHY BENEFITS OF RYE

If you love rye bread, the formidable black bread and pumpernickel Scandinavian-esque types (yes, pumpernickel is a form of rye bread), you may be doing your heart a great service. A 1996 study published in a journal of the American Heart Association suggests specifically that consuming rye bread reduces the risk of dying from heart disease. According to the study, elderly Finnish men who consumed 10 grams or more of fiber a day (about 3 slices of traditional Finnish rye) cut their risk of death from coronary heart disease by 17 percent compared to those in the study who consumed less fiber. Researchers credited fiber, especially the rye itself (which they dubbed "the wonder grain"), for being good for the heart.

Food for Thought

Rye is a "hearty" grain that's ground into flour. Denser and darker than most other flours, rye flour yields heavy loaves. Rye flour comes in various types: light, medium, dark, and pumpernickel (coarsely ground).

A Note from Dr. Jonas

TAKING CHARGE OF YOUR EATING HABITS

For many of us, taking control of our eating habits rather than having them control us is a central element in starting a healthy eating program and sticking with it. There are many choices to make: whether to change your diet at all; what goals to set; where to start. Making choices, of course, means taking responsibility for yourself. The "I'm in charge" mind-set is a very powerful psychological tool for incorporating new, positive, and healthy habits. When you're eating out or food shopping, make "I'm in charge" your mantra.

Scandinavian bread, especially the rye, barley, and other whole-grain varieties you'll find in "bread houses" and bakeries throughout Scandinavia, are no comparison to the lifeless processed rye and wheat breads we so often see in North American supermarkets. Think serious bread, the most robust rye you've ever tasted, the coarsest jaw-fatiguing whole-grain loaf you've ever chewed, and you're on the right track.

Since many North Americans consume refined, highly processed products that tend to be low in fiber, getting in 25 to 35 grams or more of fiber a day can be a tall order. Are you getting enough fiber? To find out, take this quick quiz.

1 Do you gravitate toward white bread; standard English muffins and baguettes; plain, cinnamon raisin, and other "white" bagels?
2 Do you buy cereal because it tastes good, and forgo checking the fiber content on the nutrition label?
3 Do you tend to drink fruits and vegetables (as juices) rather than eat them raw or cooked?
4 Does the thought of chopping vegetables seem like too much effort?

Answering yes to any of these questions may mean that while you think you're getting plenty of fiber, in reality, you really aren't. Eating a variety of high-fiber foods (fruits, vegetables, and whole-grain foods) is the healthiest way to boost your fiber intake. To rev up the fiber in your diet, choosing whole-grain cereals for breakfast and whole-grain breads such as whole wheat and rye like the Scandinavians do is an easy place to start. In many cases, all you'll have to do is to make slightly different food choices.

A Note from Dr. Jonas

Although a high-fiber diet can help minimize constipation in the long run, it may initially cause constipation if you consume too much fiber too soon. You may also experience diarrhea, bloating, or gas. To minimize these problems, be careful to increase your fiber intake gradually and to drink an additional glass or two of water every day. Your body will need time to adjust to the change.

The Search for Fiber

To quickly find fiber-rich breads and cereals, hunt for labels that say "good source" of fiber, which means you're getting 2.5 to 4.9 grams of fiber per serving. Even better, plop the products with labels that boast "excellent" or "high" source of fiber into your shopping cart and you'll usually get at least 5 grams of fiber per serving. To increase your fiber intake, reach for foods naturally high in fiber, such as those listed in the table below.

Some people truly like high-fiber cereals. (In Finland, a rye porridge mixed with berries is popular.) Others can't stand the taste. If you're one of the latter, try mixing a wholesome high-fiber cereal such as bran flakes with your favorite not-so-wholesome cereal. You won't even know the fiber is there. Also, when buying whole-grain breads in North America, look for the key word "whole"—as in "whole wheat," "whole grain," and "whole oats"—as the first ingredient on the label. Products described as "wheat" (minus "whole") don't cut it. Without the operative word "whole," you may simply be buying a product made with white flour since white flour is made from wheat. And keep in mind that "multigrain" or "7-grain" can also be code words for fiber-deficient bread as well.

And finally, you might try topping casseroles with whole-grain cereal and using crushed whole-grain cereal instead of white flour as a coating for chicken.

Whole-Grain High-Fiber Favorites

FOOD	SERVING SIZE	CALORIES	FIBER (GRAMS)
North American–style rye bread	1 slice	83	2
Whole-grain bread	1 slice	105	3
Brown rice	1 cup, cooked	220	3
Whole-wheat bread	1 slice	105	3
Oatmeal	1 cup, cooked	300	9
Raisin bran with skim milk	1 cup cereal with ½ cup milk	240	8
Fat-free raisin bran muffin	1 medium	100	9
Barley	½ cup, cooked	190	9
Extra-Fiber All Bran with skim milk	½ cup cereal with ½ cup skim milk	90	13

Food for Thought

Why are whole-grain breads and cereals so popular in the Scandinavian countries? In many cases, Mother Nature dictates. Especially in Finland and Denmark, stalwart sourdough rye and barley bread rule because the growing season isn't long enough to permit wheat to mature. Norway, on the other hand, imports wheat flour, so more wheat bread is available there; and Sweden is able to grow its own wheat. Still, the end result is a health-promoting coarse wheat bread, what the Norwegians and Swedes call "whole-meal bread," not the processed wheat and "light" rye breads with which North Americans are more familiar.

Food for Thought

To spot high-fiber foods in Swedish supermarkets, Swedish consumers look for grain and bread products with a green key-hole symbol on the label. This symbol means that the product has whole grains among its in-gredients and is a good source of fiber. At least half the number of cereals on Sweden's supermarket shelves sport green keyholes. Incidentally, Sweden and the United States are the only countries to have national uniform food-labeling programs to help consumers make healthier food-purchasing decisions.

GLOBAL EATING SECRET #25

Switch to Skim or 1 or 2 Percent Milk

The people of Scandinavia are some of the world's most famous dairy lovers. Jukka Oresto, the Finnish food journalist, says that in Finland, "there is al-ways milk on the table when families have their meal. Even in restaurants, people have milk with their dinner." (Of course, he adds, many people also drink water, wine, or beer.)

Maybe you've been meaning to switch from whole milk to 2 percent fat, or 2 percent to nonfat milk, from ice cream to low-fat frozen yogurt. But you just can't quite make the swap. You'll be giving up too much flavor, won't you? Need motivation? Enter the Scandinavians and the Finns, formerly the world's biggest consumers of full-fat dairy products, the kind laden with artery-clogging saturated fat.

For decades, the peoples of Nordic countries consumed a diet loaded with high-fat dairy products such as butter, whole-fat cheese, whole milk, and cream, known as "squeezed milk." In Finland, for example, where the rates of heart disease soared untethered from 1940 to 1970, "they were enormous milk drinkers," says Elizabeth Helsing, Ph.D., of the international section of the Norwegian Board of Health. They'd typically down a glass of whole milk for breakfast and another at lunch. They'd spread a thick layer of butter on a couple of slices of rye bread, slap them together, and call the result a sand-wich. They'd douse their numerous daily cups of boiled coffee with cream. After dinner, they'd relax with a dish of berry cream, a milky sweet dessert. These fat-dense dairy products were simply part of their culinary culture be-cause that was what was available. (Dairy farmers were in on the deal; they made fatter profits by producing high-fat dairy products.)

Eventually, however, Scandinavian dairy farmers came around (with a nudge by the government) and began producing low-fat dairy items. Mean-while, nationwide government food policies were instituted to encourage consumers in Denmark, Sweden, Finland, and Norway to buy these low-fat products for their health.

While many Scandinavian consumers are buying low-fat dairy products, others are cutting back on dairy products entirely. "People are more conscious about the effects of healthy eating. They're beginning to realize that we have a rich cooking tradition to fall back on in Finland—if we just cut down on our consumption of butter and cream," says Maria Planting, a chef at the Hel-sinki Culinary Institute. In Denmark, they're learning to prepare traditional specialties such as *frikadeller* (Swedish meatballs) made from a blend of beef, pork, and veal and topped with a sauce, sans the cream. And when it comes to bread, "it's becoming a trend not to butter it," says Tove Færch, head of Caroline's Kitchen, the recipe development arm of the Danish Dairy Board in Copenhagen.

As noted, epidemiologists attest that it's no coincidence that the rates of heart disease in Scandinavia have fallen drastically in recent years and continue to decline. If the Scandinavians can learn to love low-fat and nonfat dairy products, anyone can.

Got Fat-Free Milk?

North Americans are ahead of the game. Our supermarkets have been offering low-fat dairy products for years. More recently, nonfat dairy products have come on the scene. Still, to reduce the saturated fat in your meals (and reduce your risk of heart disease), it pays to be choosy. The low-fat and nonfat dairy options in your market, in coffee bars, and in restaurants are often surrounded by an abundance of high-fat ones. Here are your best bets for cutting the fat in your diet from dairy products:

- Opt for nonfat yogurt. Just 1 cup provides 240 milligrams of calcium (almost one-fourth of the 1,000 to 1,500 milligram recommended dietary allowance for calcium) and zero fat.

- Switch to nonfat (skim) milk. If you think skim milk tastes watery, try different brands. Many now have added milk solids that give the "mouth feel" of 2 percent milk. Guaranteed, your taste buds will be fooled.

- Put 2 percent milk—not cream—in your coffee, and you'll save nearly 4 grams of fat and 30 fat calories per tablespoon. (Go ahead and ask for milk for your coffee at restaurants that keep cream ready and waiting on the table.)

- Switch to "skinny" caffè lattes (made with skim milk). This standard pick-me-up at coffee bars can offer a significant source of calcium without the fat (you won't miss it).

- Reach for nonfat cottage cheese, which is made from skim milk, rather than the brands with 4 percent milkfat. Just ½ cup of delicious nonfat cottage cheese provides 10 percent of the recommended daily dietary allowance for calcium and zero fat.

- Substitute plain nonfat yogurt for the same amount of mayonnaise in a recipe. Tablespoon per tablespoon, you'll save 90 calories and nearly 12 grams of fat. You'll be hard-pressed to detect a taste difference.

The Health Benefits of Calcium

No doubt, you know that being a dairy devotee like the people of Scandinavia and getting plenty of calcium is one of the best ways to ward off bone-thinning osteoporosis later in life. But that's not all. The latest research from international and national studies shows that there are new reasons to make sure your calcium intake meets the recommended amount—1,000 milligrams a day for adults (1,200 to 1,500 mg if you're pregnant or nursing). Here are just a few of the benefits, besides stronger bones, that you'll reap from a low-fat, calcium-rich diet.

- **Beating breast cancer.** Besides helping prevent bone loss, calcium may also help reduce the risk of breast cancer, especially if you're a milk drinker. A Finnish study involving over 4,600 women concluded that those who drank about three 8-ounce glasses of milk a day had the lowest risk of breast cancer compared to those who didn't drink that amount. In fairness, however, calcium can't take all the credit. Researchers suspect that conjugated linoleic acid (CLA), a type of fat found in milk, may also have potent cancer-fighting properties.

- **Combating colon cancer.** As mentioned earlier, colon cancer—the uncontrolled growth of abnormal cells in the colon—

A Note from Dr. Jonas
FINDING YOUR FOOTING

Achieving balance is an important part of sticking with a pattern of healthy eating. To be a healthy eater over a lifetime doesn't always mean eating only so-called healthy foods. It doesn't mean never having a juicy steak or never having a hot fudge sundae again. It simply means cutting down on the frequency with which, among other things, less-than-optimal foods appear in your diet. Once you get to a point in which you're eating foods that have a lot to offer nutritionally, it's entirely okay to indulge on occasion.

Once you get used to eating healthier, however, I'll venture to guess that you'll come to seek out these kinds of foods. Your palate will change. Milk, for example, will taste funny unless it's fat-free. A vegetable-light meal will seem like it's missing something. You'll feel the effects when you don't eat as well as you normally do. But that's not to say that you won't have that slice of cheesecake now and then. After all, an occasional treat can be psychologically healthy, helping you avoid feelings of deprivation.

is one of the most commonly diagnosed cancers in men and women in the United States. Recent studies show that a diet rich in calcium may help prevent this invasive disease. The theory: Without adequate calcium, bile and fatty acids— natural by-products of digestion—can irritate cells lining the colon, leading to a state in which cells are constantly undergoing repair. This increases the likelihood that these cells may become cancerous. The more cells regenerate, the more their DNA (a cell's message center) has the opportunity of being hit with toxic agents, which can cause them to divide too rapidly. Calcium, however, binds with these pesky acids in the colon, possibly preventing them from doing damage.

- **Downsizing PMS.** Women: With more calcium in your diet, you're apt to suffer less from the mood swings, headaches, smoldering irritability, and jittery anxiety associated with that time of the month. A major study from St. Luke's Roosevelt Hospital in New York City showed that a daily dose of 1,200 to 1,500 milligrams of calcium can reduce those classic PMS signs by 50 percent. The study concluded that premenstrual symptoms are an indication of an underlying calcium deficiency as well as a sign of probable bone loss, since it's thought that the same hormones regulate both conditions.

- **Preventing high blood pressure.** As discussed earlier in this book, high blood pressure can lead to heart disease, the

A Note from Dr. Jonas
SIZING UP YOUR SUPPLEMENT

In an ideal world, it's best to get your calcium from food because it contains a complete package of nutrients that may help fight disease. Yet, it's estimated that 30 to 50 percent of North American women, for example, get less than the recommended calcium intakes. (You could be one of them if you frequently drink diet soda, for example, instead of low-fat or fat-free milk at meals.) If this sounds like you, consider taking a calcium supplement for added health insurance. (If you have a personal or family medical history of kidney stones, however, first talk to your doctor.)

If you go the supplement route, use it to top off the calcium you get from your diet. Strive for 500 milligrams of calcium a day from a supplement and get the remaining 500 to 1,000 milligrams of calcium from food.

Calcium supplements come in different forms such as calcium gluconate, Tums (calcium carbonate), and calcium citrate. Because all are absorbed more or less equally well, your main concern when choosing a supplement and estimating how many supplements you need to take each day is how much pure, elemental calcium your supplement contains. Finding out is easy—just look on the Nutrition Facts panel on the label. Moreover, to make sure your body absorbs the maximum amount of calcium from your supplement, heed these ground rules:

Take it with meals. Because food helps slow the rate at which calcium is absorbed in your intestine, taking a calcium supplement with food, preferably with larger meals, increases by 10 to 15 percent the amount of calcium your body will take from a supplement.

Divide and conquer. Spread your supplement intake out in several doses. For example, if you're taking 500 milligrams of calcium a day, take 250 milligrams at lunch and another 250 milligrams at dinner to increase the number of times your intestine is exposed to calcium. (You might do this by taking a multivitamin-multimineral supplement with calcium at lunch, and then taking a straight calcium supplement at dinner.)

Aim for a name brand. Compared with store brands and small-time manufacturers, brand-name supplement makers generally have more knowledge and experience—and a professional reputation to protect. You may pay a little more for a name-brand supplement, but you'll gain greater confidence that you're buying a quality calcium product your body will absorb.

Choose a calcium supplement with vitamin D. Vitamin D helps fine-tune calcium absorption. This is especially important as you get older. With age, many people synthesize less vitamin D from the sun and other sources.

leading cause of death for both men and women in the United States. High blood pressure during pregnancy—a condition called preeclampsia—is also a formidable health threat.

Calcium from dairy products, however, in combination with a balanced, low-fat diet may help keep blood pressure in check. In a major study called DASH (Dietary Approaches to Stop Hypertension) conducted by, among others, researchers from the National Heart, Lung, and Blood Institute, calcium was one of several nutrients in high amounts that lowered blood pressure. In fact, out of the DASH study came the official DASH diet, which is similar to the USDA Food Pyramid, to prevent and control high blood pressure. The DASH diet, which is widely distributed to high blood pressure patients in the United States, recommends two to three servings daily of low-fat or nonfat calcium-rich dairy foods such as skim milk, nonfat yogurt, and low-fat cheese.

Food for thought

The Danish diet dichotomy: In Denmark, the general tendency is to "be good" during the week—to skip the butter, layer bread with low-fat cheese, and eat more fruits and vegetables. But on the weekends, look out. "We have a Danish expression that means we have to take good care of ourselves. It's okay to be a little unhealthy. To have your time to be relaxed and do what

• **Putting the kibosh on kidney stones.** Women: If you've ever had a kidney stone, you know those minute collections of minerals that form in the kidneys can cause excruciating pain if they attempt to pass through the urinary tract and out of the body. Most kidney stones are made from calcium and oxalate, a saltlike substance found in foods such as beets, spinach, rhubarb, and nuts. Your body also steadily makes its own oxalate supply. Normally, calcium and oxalate remain dissolved and are excreted in the urine. But stones can form when calcium and oxalate become too concentrated in the kidneys, becoming a solid not unlike sugar settling to the bottom of your coffee cup. A 12-year Harvard study involving over 90,000 women, however, found that those with the highest calcium intake had the lowest risk of kidney stones. The theory? Calcium binds with oxalate during digestion, canceling out the possibility that stones will form down the pike. A caveat: The same study also showed that taking calcium supplements *without* food may actually increase the likelihood that kidney stones will form in some people.

Making the Calcium Connection

To help meet the recommended calcium intake of 1,000 to 1,500 milligrams a day, strive to consume at least three low-fat or nonfat calcium-rich foods daily, such as those in the table below.

If you're lactose intolerant, suggesting that your body lacks an enzyme that helps digest lactose, a carbohydrate found in milk, try consuming dairy foods such as milk, cheese, or yogurt *with* meals. Food slows the rate lactose enters your intestine so your body can handle it better. Lactose-free milk and cottage cheese (called "HYLA products" in Finland) are also other options, as is soy milk, but make sure it's calcium fortified with at least 30 percent of the daily value (check the label).

Low-fat and Nonfat Sources of Calcium

FOOD	SERVING SIZE	CALORIES	CALCIUM (MILLIGRAMS)	ADDED BONUS
Low-fat or non-fat yogurt	1 cup	210/100	350/400	Contains active cultures, which helps make yogurt especially digestible if you're lactose intolerant.
Fat-free (skim) milk	1 cup	90	250	One of the easiest ways to get more calcium. Swap water or soda for skim milk at meals; make oatmeal, canned soups, pancakes from a mix, and prepared cake mixes with milk instead of water; order a skinny latte (⅔ skim milk, ⅓ espresso) instead of regular coffee at coffee bars.

you like. To use cream if you want to. To eat Danish pastry instead of rye bread. To stack your open-faced sandwich [a Danish institution] with meats and cheeses. This applies to the weekend," says Tove Færch of the Danish Dairy Board. Moreover, according to Lars Ovesen, the contributor to the chapter on Denmark in Implementing Dietary Guidelines for Healthy Eating, "it's a common belief that healthy food is more expensive, takes more time to prepare, and is less tasty than unhealthy food." Not surprisingly, Denmark has experienced only a modest improvement in life expectancy in recent years compared to most other European countries.

FOOD	SERVING SIZE	CALORIES	CALCIUM (MILLIGRAMS)	ADDED BONUS
Fat-free, lactose-free milk	1 cup	90	300	A good substitute for regular milk.
Fat-free frozen yogurt	½ cup	100	450	The best brands provide 45 percent of the daily value for calcium (check the label)—more calcium than in a glass of milk.
Lowfat ice cream	½ cup	120	150	Contains a fraction of the fat and calories of regular ice cream.
Calcium-fortified orange or grapefruit juice	1 cup	120/100	350	A glass of either has more than a full day's supply of the antioxidant vitamin C; oj is also a good source of folate.
Low-fat cheese such as mozzarella	1" cube	50	150	Half the fat of regular mozzarella.
Calcium-fortified cottage cheese	½ cup	80	200	A good source of protein; twice the calcium of regular cottage cheese.
Firm tofu	⅛ block	50	150	Firm tofu offers nearly 10 percent more calcium than soft varieties.
Salmon (with bones)	¼ cup	90	100	Easy to incorporate into your diet—substitute for tuna in a sandwich on occasion.

Fat Track Record

In the traditional Scandinavian diet, the saturated fat from butter, meat, milk, and cheese contributed nearly the entire fat intake due to the wide availability of these products. Fortunately, thanks to development of low-fat dairy products, fat consumption is decreasing, rivaling the amount of fat we're consuming in North America. Look how well they've done:

- In 1985, average Danes got 44 percent of their calories from fat (10 percent more than the average North American gets now). By the late 1990s, however, fat consumption was down to 37 percent.
- In Finland, between 1982 and 1992, the total fat content of the Finnish diet declined from 38 percent of energy to 34 percent.
- During a similar time span, fat intake dropped from 37 to 35 percent of total calories in Sweden.
- Between 1970 and the late 1990s, fat consumption in Norway decreased from 40 percent to 34 percent.

The Swedish Plate Special

To encourage Swedish consumers to eat more fruits and vegetables as well as fiber-rich grains, Swedish government officials developed "the plate model," which is equivalent to the USDA Food Pyramid. The bread and grains and fruit and vegetable sections take up three-fourths of the plate; the meat, fish, and eggs section accounts for the rest.

――――――― G L O B A L   E A T I N G   S E C R E T   # 26 ―――――――
Eat More Green Foods

From the beginning, this book has been singing the praises of eating more fruits and vegetables. North Americans just don't get enough of this magic and powerful disease-fighting food group. But here's something to make you feel better, if only temporarily: The Scandinavians eat fewer servings of produce a day than we do. In fact, fruits and vegetables really aren't part of their

---

A Note from Dr. Jonas
TAKE SEVERAL STEPS TO GUARD AGAINST OSTEOPOROSIS

Even though Scandinavians are famous for their milk drinking, osteoporosis is still a threat to them. Contributing factors include the lack of sunlight (and thus lack of bone-building vitamin D), the lack of exercise (yes, even the hearty Nordics need to exercise more), and the fact that more Scandinavian women are taking up smoking. (Smoking is linked to an increased risk of osteoporosis.) Moreover, high doses of caffeine (remember their copious coffee consumption?) can cause the body to lose small amounts of calcium.

Food for Thought

Eating more fruit, vegetables, and fiber can help you lower your cholesterol. But more margarine? If it hasn't already, Benecol, a big seller in Finland where it was invented, is soon to hit supermarket shelves in your area. This margarine-like spread contains wood pulp extract that is purported to reduce cholesterol levels by 10 percent—without making any other changes in your diet. The secret to Benecol is sitostanol, a pine extract that helps block some dietary cholesterol from being absorbed in the *intestines where it enters the bloodstream. In Finland, the invention of Benecol did more than make people aware of the national cholesterol problem. It triggered an intensive publicity campaign about healthier eating habits. Now, most consumers there know to reduce their consumption of butter, cream, and whole milk. Still, "old habits die hard," says Helsinki chef Maria Planting. Benecol is just one of the many "functional" foods to hit store shelves in Finland. Among others is a sausage that helps lower cholesterol.*

Food for Thought

Although much of the fish harvested from Scandinavia's coastline and its famous fiords is exported, Scandinavian consumers are consummate fish eaters who are fond of reeling their fish in right from local icy waters, thus making them reluctant to buy fish in markets and restaurants. On the Nordic table, you'll frequently find Baltic herring, laks

culinary tradition. In the past, the quality, selection, and quantity of fruits and vegetables we take for granted simply wasn't available in Scandinavian food markets. In Norway, this is still the case. A typical supermarket produce section "is a sad sight," says Dr. Helsing, of the Norwegian Board of Health. Still, fruit and vegetable consumption in Norway has increased two- to three-fold between 1982 and 1992 because availability is improving slightly and consumers are experimenting with the new supply. For example, "twenty years ago, we would not touch the strange-looking vegetables called bell peppers," says Dr. Helsing. "Now, they're part of the diet."

In other Scandinavian countries, they're enjoying North American–style bounty. In Sweden, for example, produce sections of supermarkets, once limited to apples, oranges, bananas, and cold-weather vegetables such as cabbage and potatoes, now display a wide variety of produce year-round, including exotic options such as mangoes, papayas, and kiwifruit. Because of influence from the Mediterranean and the Caribbean, "we have at least forty different fruits and vegetables to choose from," boasts Birgitta Rasmusson, a test-kitchen manager at ICA, a publishing house in Stockholm. In Stockholm, a particularly progressive metropolis, "green eating" is also popular. That is, dining at restaurants that offer "legume burgers" and other strictly vegetarian fare, a wholly novel concept to this part of the world.

Getting More Fruits and Vegetables the Scandinavian Way

The average North American major supermarket typically offers more than a hundred kinds of fruits and vegetables no matter what season of the year. As mentioned throughout this book, fruits and vegetables are a great source of fiber, vitamins, minerals, and phytochemicals that can help you fight diseases such as cancer and heart disease. Are you making the most of this opportunity? To get in the habit of consuming five to nine servings of fruits and vegetables a day as recommended by the National Cancer Institute, here are three Scandinavian-inspired suggestions that you could easily import into your routine:

- **Fortify your salad.** For years, a Swedish salad consisted of lettuce, tomato, and cucumber. But now, the Swedes are taking full advantage of the plethora of produce on the market and topping their standard salads off with such items as chopped bell peppers, onions, mushrooms, beets, and grated carrots. To save chopping time, they're buying the precut, prepackaged vegetables and greens now also available to North Americans.

- **Serve berries for dessert.** Wild berry desserts have always been a Scandinavian tradition, especially those made with lingonberries, a member of the cranberry family that grows in the mountains of Scandinavia. Served au natural, or stewed and thickened with flour, lingonberries aren't widely available in North America. No matter. For a quick hit after dinner or for a snack, who can resist popular North American standbys such as fresh blueberries, raspberries, or strawberries? All happen to be excellent sources of vitamin C, a potent antioxidant. You might also try pureeing raspberries with a little sugar and dolloping this healthy sauce on top of low-fat or nonfat vanilla frozen yogurt. (Don't strain the seeds. They're a good source of fiber and offer a delightful crunch.) Homemade raspberry sauce (instead of syrup) also makes a delicious and nutritious topping for pancakes, waffles, and French toast.

- **Stack your sandwich.** The traditional Denmark version of the open-face sandwich (*smørrebrød*), offered at the grandest of restaurants to the lowliest of pushcarts, resembles a leaning tower that's been known to have a layer of anything from cucumber to peaches. The next time you go the sandwich route, use it as an opportunity to layer in sliced fruits and vegetables Danish-style: lettuce, tomatoes, cucumbers, bell pepper, onion, apples. Their motto: If you can slice it, you can stack it.

(salmon), and makrel *(mackerel), smoked and otherwise. Of course, these fatty fish offer liberal amounts of omega-3 fatty acids, the good-for-you fat discussed at length in the Mediterranean chapter.*

Food for Thought

As in the United States and other countries, the governments of Scandinavia are encouraging citizens to eat more produce to protect against cancer. In Denmark, for example, the government is running a "six-a-day" campaign, lobbying for consumers to double their fruit and vegetable consumption and eat six servings of fruits or vegetables daily.

WESTERN AFRICA
Foods for Cancer Protection

We thank Thee Almighty God
For giving us Cassava
We hail Thee Cassava
The Great Cassava
We shall sing your praise.

—Flora Nwapa, from the
"Cassava Song" as quoted
from *Fighting Hunger with
Cassava*, African Action on
AIDS

To conclude our culinary journey to the lands of the world's healthiest diets, we're venturing southwest to The Gambia, the smallest country on the continent of Africa. For years, during the cool, dry season from November through June, tourists have flocked to The Gambia's luxury hotels in search of an affordable yet exotic respite. This country's glorious sunshine, piercing blue skies, friendly people, and 200-plus species of birds and other wildlife draw scores of sun-seekers, adventurers, and nature lovers annually. But perhaps tour operators should also promote the local cuisine, because The Gambia (this country's official name in honor of the Gambia River, which flows through this agrarian village of 1 million people) has a hidden health secret: Cancer rates are the lowest in the world.

Indeed, despite its high incidence rates of potentially deadly communicable diseases such as malaria and HIV, The Gambia has the lowest rate of breast cancer in the world, even lower than Japan's. According to statistics published by the U.S. National Institutes of Health, The Gambia reports the lowest overall incidence of cancer for any country in the world.

How do these tribal village people manage to live so cancer free? It's likely their diet has something to do with it. The Gambian diet is essentially plant based, with only a nod to meat. As you likely know by now, a regular regime of mostly vegetables, fruit, and grains provides disease protection in the form of nutrients, antioxidants, phytochemicals, and fiber that may short-circuit the cellular processes that lead to cancer. A plant-based diet is considered especially cancer protective when coupled with high levels of physical activity. As it stands, roughly 75 percent of Gambians depend on some form of hands-on agriculture for their livelihood, activity that no doubt contributes to The Gambia's low rate of obesity. But you don't have to trek thousands of miles to far corners of the world to experience this international incident firsthand. Here's how to fight cancer the Gambian way by traveling only as far as your local supermarket.

The Gambia at a Glance

Low rates of breast and other cancers

• The Gambia has the lowest rates of breast cancer in the world, even lower than Japan's. Moreover, The Gambia reports the lowest international incidence of all types of cancer.

A meat-light diet

• Vegetable-based stews dominate the Gambian diet.

• Among a host of vegetables, yams are a Gambian staple. Although not widely sold in North America, their even healthier cousin, the sweet potato, is available year-round. Sweet potatoes are an excellent source of the antioxidant vitamins A and C as well as fat-free carbohydrates. When it comes to disease protection, they're a power food.

Food hot enough to match the climate

• Gambians don't shy away from spicy food, thanks to the hot peppers that flourish there, soaking up some of the sun's sizzle. Spicy food won't speed up your metabolism, but it can jazz up a healthy diet.

GLOBAL EATING SECRET #27

Stew Your Foods

A slew of stews is one of the hallmarks of Gambian cuisine, especially if you're a member of the Wolof and Mandinka tribes, which comprise over 50 percent of the Gambian population. Spicy, vegetable-based concoctions, perhaps flavored with bits of fish, beef, cow's hooves, goat, or oxtail, top the list of classic Gambian tribal recipes. On any traditional Gambian restaurant menu, for example, you're likely to find *domoda*—peanut-and-tomato-based stew with cubes of beef *(nak)*. You'll also spot *yasa*—cabbage, carrots, and onions with garlic sauce and perhaps a bit of chicken *(cope)* as well as *soupe-au-kanja*—beef, okra, and spinach in ginger sauce—all of which are served over a steaming bowl of rice. *Thiebujin,* a jambalaya-esque fish dish is also a popular Gambian specialty.

We North Americans tend to beef up our stew with loads of beef chuck or beef round. But stews—technically any dish prepared with a combination of vegetables and meat in a thick souplike broth and simmered leisurely—are a flavorful way to get a variety of vegetables into your diet without even realizing it. (In The Gambia, stews are also a necessary meat stretcher, since meat is expensive and availability is limited.)

To minimize the meat content of your diet and maximize your vegetable intake, consider serving stews and stewlike dishes more often. To enhance their cancer-fighting properties, however, prepare them the Gambian way: Take the opportunity to throw in as many vegetables as you can stand. Vegetable combinations Gambians often favor include onions, tomatoes, carrots, potatoes, cabbage, eggplant, plantains, yams, lima and butter beans, okra, gourd, pumpkin, and squash.

GLOBAL EATING SECRET #28
Vary Your Potatoes

As mentioned in earlier chapters, North Americans love potatoes, which would be a favorable fact if we'd eat them naked and baked. A 3.5-ounce baked white potato with the skin—sans the butter, sour cream, or gravy—offers more potassium (beneficial for keeping blood pressure in check) than a 6-ounce glass of orange juice, only 110 calories, and no fat. Baked potatoes also contain good amounts of iron, vitamin C, and energizing carbohydrates. Unfortunately, the majority of potatoes in North America are likely to end up fried, a preparation method that ups their calorie and fat count per ounce considerably, making them a less-than-optimal option.

Good News about the Sweet Potato

Enter the Gambians. An everyday vegetable in western Africa is the yam, a sizeable cousin to our sweet potato. In western Africa, yams *(fu-fu)* balloon

Food for Thought

The idea that a high-fiber diet protects against colon cancer originated in Africa when researchers found that Africans who ate diets very high in fiber had a low incidence of colon cancer compared with the rest of the world.

up to 100 pounds and are traditionally "pounded" with a mortar and pestle after they've been boiled, and then molded into a cake and sliced.

Most sweet potatoes—both fresh and canned—in stores in North America are called "yams," but technically, yams aren't widely available here. But, of course, we can buy sweet potatoes year-round, which is all the better. If you're trying to infuse your diet with more disease-fighting power, keep the sweet potato in mind.

Thanks to its superior nutrient portfolio, the sweet potato is the CEO of vegetables. Consider this: The sweet potato offers vast amounts of the antioxidant vitamin A (the true yam, incidentally, has none) and is a stellar source of vitamin C, potassium, and fiber, which, as mentioned earlier, may help protect against colon and other cancers as well as heart disease and high blood pressure. A high-fiber diet may also help prevent and manage Type 2 diabetes. Moreover, a 3.5-ounce baked sweet potato contains only 105 calories and no fat. No doubt, it's one of the most nutrient-dense choices in the vegetable kingdom.

Rather than simply reserving sweet potatoes for holidays such as Thanksgiving, consider substituting them for white potatoes whenever you have the chance. Bake fresh sweet potatoes and serve them hot or cold, in the skin, with a little brown sugar if needed for flavoring. Canned sweet potatoes, skinless and packed in syrup, are a less healthful choice.

For an African Twist—Consider the Cassava

Alongside the yam, the cassava, a starchy tuber with a nutlike flavor, grows abundantly in western Africa without much prodding. It is also called *manioc*, and is the source of tapioca. Noted for its perseverance, endurance, and survival instinct, the cassava sports a woody brown bark, beneath which lies a creamy white interior. The cassava often measures 1 foot long and weighs up to 3 pounds, the size of a child-size football. Maybe you've eyed the cassava in your supermarket's "exotic" fruit and vegetable section or at your local Latin or Asian market.

A good source of vitamin C, potassium, iron, and fat-free carbohydrates, the cassava has only 120 calories per 3.5-ounce serving. It's in-

---

A Note from Dr. Jonas
THE LIMITS OF THE GAMBIAN DIET

Although the high-fiber yams and the other vegetables in the Gambian diet may help reduce the risk of high blood pressure, this so-called silent killer is as prevalent in The Gambia as it is among many African Americans in the United States. In this case, as with any disease or condition, genetic makeup is likely a contributing factor.

cluded here not because it's nutritionally superior to the baked white potato (it isn't), but because it's another way to introduce international interest into your diet. To make a healthy diet more intriguing, why not venture abroad in the produce aisle and occasionally try the cassava instead of potatoes? To prepare the cassava, simply peel the bark and underlayer, slice the crisp, white flesh in chunks, and cook thoroughly in a small amount of water as you would white potatoes. Serve it mashed or boiled; it's also a suitable, occasional substitute for regular potatoes in soups and stews.

------------ GLOBAL EATING SECRET #29 ------------

Turn Up the Heat

Some like it hot, and this is especially true in The Gambia. "Ooh, I still love that hot pepper," says a reminiscent Juliana Rowe, a native of western Africa who has lived in New York City for several years. In The Gambia, for example, high-Fahrenheit sauces prepared with pungent cayenne pepper and a handful of hot chilis infuse countless native dishes, igniting a lurking smolder.

Contrary to popular belief, spicy foods don't boost your metabolism, the rate at which you burn calories. (To shift your metabolism into high gear, exercise is your best bet. For each pound of muscle you gain, you'll burn roughly 35 more calories per day.) But spicy foods may help you get more enjoyment out of eating a lower-fat diet. By firing up your meals, you'll be less apt to miss butter, cream sauces, and that crispy coating. Moreover, research suggests that the slightly discomforting sensation that heat produces may also cause the brain to release endorphins. These feel-good neurotransmitters are associated with the "runner's high" that exercisers tend to get after a lengthy workout. Spicy foods are an acquired taste. Nonetheless, it pays to be a risk taker. With a moment of gustatory pain, there's often pleasure.

A Note from Dr. Jonas
THE MYTH OF SPICY FOODS

Contrary to an old wives' tale, spicy foods won't give you ulcers. Nor will a bland diet heal them. Recent studies show that *Helicobacter pylori,* a bacteria that burrows into your stomach, is the real culprit behind most peptic or esophageal ulcers—irritations or sores that occur in the lining of the stomach, the duodenum (part of the small intestine), or the esophagus. Instead of a bland diet, antibiotics are now the standard ulcer therapy. If you think you may have an ulcer, see your doctor. Classic symptoms: a burning feeling in the stomach about forty-five minutes to two hours after eating, or frequent abdominal pain that's goes away after eating, drinking milk, or taking an antacid.

GLOBAL EATING SECRET #30

Eat More Peanuts

In western Africa, peanuts are a "cash crop," a valuable commodity produced for market on which, for example, the Gambian economy is based. You'll find peanuts boiled and roasted as well as featured in soups and a classic Gambian entrée called *domoda*, commonly known as "ground nut stew." This peanut butter stew features chunks of onions, tomatoes, chicken, and pumpkin heaped over rice. You'll also find leaves with dollops of peanut butter sold in Gambian markets.

A generous handful of dry-roasted peanuts packs 160 calories and a hefty 13 grams of fat. For years, registered dietitians and other nutrition professionals have been training consumers who are trying to lose weight to run from the nut dish at parties and to spread a mere sheer veil of peanut butter on toast. Recent studies suggest, however, that all this energy spent avoiding the consequences of peanut consumption may have been wasted—that peanuts are good for you, and can even be a part of a sensible weight-loss plan.

Something Nutty

One such preliminary study conducted at Pennsylvania State University found that a diet that contained 35 percent of calories as fat, but contained peanuts and peanut butter as well as other foods high in heart-healthy monounsaturated fat, didn't stop participants from losing 2 pounds a week over a six-week period. The study concluded that a diet high in monounsaturated fat is as good as a low-fat diet for weight loss as long as calorie intake is controlled.

During an eighteen-month weight-loss study at Harvard Medical School and Brigham and Women's Hospital in Boston, 101 overweight men and women were assigned to follow either a low-fat diet or one higher in monounsaturated fat. Almost three times as many people were able to stick to a higher-fat diet that included peanuts and peanut butter than could stick to a lower-fat one. Moreover, compared with the peanut eaters, those on the low-fat diet gained back most of the weight they lost—roughly 11 pounds.

Beyond their judicious role in a sensible weight-loss plan, peanuts have also been shown to be good for you for reasons other than that they contain a higher percentage of cholesterol-busting, heart-healthy monounsaturated fat.

Food for Thought

In western Africa, which is 90 percent Muslim, religious custom dictates that left-handers may be at a disadvantage. "Using your left hand to eat is taboo, as is handing someone food—or anything for that matter—with your left hand," says Justice Matey, a chef at the Bukon Café, a West African restaurant in the Adams Morgan section of Washington, D.C. A left-handed offering is considered bad manners and a blatant display of disrespect, particularly if you're giving something with your left hand to an elder.

They're a good source of B vitamins, including folate (the food form of folic acid); protein; iron; fiber; and vitamin E, higher intakes of which are associated with a lower risk of heart disease. Peanuts have also been found to contain the phytochemical resveratrol, the heart-disease-fighting substance also identified in red wine.

And consider this: Peanuts have also been shown to contain phytoesterols, the plant version of cholesterol. (Cholesterol, of course, is only found in animal-based foods such as butter, cream, meat, and eggs.) One phytoesterol in particular, beta-sitosterol (SIT), which is prevalent in peanuts and peanut products, has been found to inhibit cancer growth, a factor that may contribute to the low cancer incidence rate in The Gambia. When it comes to eating globally, an ever increasing body of research supports the theory that eating peanuts isn't such a nutty idea.

Watch Out for Tropical Oils

The traditional Gambian diet isn't perfect. Although more Gambians are discovering vegetable and olive oils and trying to eat a lower-fat diet, many still make traditional Gambian recipes with palm oil, a reddish-orange oil from the pulp of the fruit of a native African palm. One dish mentioned earlier, *soupe-au-kanja*, for example, is otherwise known as "okra palm oil stew." An acquired taste, palm oil is by no means hidden. When used in cooking, "it colors everything red," says Juliana Rowe, a native of Sierra Leone, the African country known for its rebel wars, which also happens to share a cuisine similar to The Gambia.

On a par with animal fats such as butter and lard, so-called tropical oils like palm, palm kernel, and coconut are high in artery-clogging saturated fat. But because they add texture and flavor to foods and are a relatively inexpensive ingredient, you'll frequently find them in processed and snack foods sold in North America. Many Gambians may be physically active enough to

---

A Note from Dr. Jonas

HELP FOR THOSE ALLERGIC TO PEANUTS

According to the American Academy of Allergy, Asthma, and Immunology, approximately 3 million Americans are allergic to nuts, including peanuts. If you suspect that you're one of them, you'll of course want to avoid peanuts. But because an allergic reaction to nuts can be fatal, you should also be prepared to self-treat a peanut allergy should you have a reaction. Peanuts, after all, are one of the most popular nuts in America and are served on airplanes and sold widely in countless places. People with an allergy to nuts are often advised to carry a small dose of self-administering epinephrine, which can halt the attack. If you think you might be subject to such an attack, talk to your doctor for more information.

Food for Thought

At one time, plumpness in women in traditionally poor western Africa was a sign of wealth. "It showed that you were well fed and that your husband could afford you," says Banusi Jallow, a South African married to a Gambian. The goal was to give form to your boo boo, a traditional African gown with an interior wraparound skirt. "A boo boo is long and homey. You had to fill it out so people could still see your body shape. Other-

wise, you looked like you were suffering," Ms. Jallow says. Fortunately, with more Gambians traveling now and learning other ways of life, being overweight in The Gambia is no longer considered a status symbol.

compensate for a diet that features this saturated fat, but the average North American isn't. To discover what products contain these saturated fats, get into the habit of reading food labels, especially on processed foods. To reduce your risk of heart disease, obesity, and other conditions, it's a good idea to limit, or better yet, avoid products that list palm, palm kernel, or coconut oils on their labels.

8

The Global Eating Menu Plan
for Weight Maintenance or Weight Loss

This chapter features the Global Eating Menu Plan, which is designed to help you truly begin importing into your diet the best eating habits from the countries and regions discussed throughout this book.

This one-week megahealthy menu plan can help you begin reaping the health benefits of the world's healthiest diets by taking your eating habits in a new, more adventurous, and tastier direction. Developed by Courtney Gravenese, a registered dietitian and exercise physiologist in New York City, the Global Eating Menu Plan includes a 2,000-calorie version for those who wish to maintain their weight, and a 1,500-calorie plan for those who want to lose 1 to 2 pounds a week, with suggestions for how to vary each diet if you choose to follow either indefinitely.

Rest assured that neither menu plan will require that you completely overhaul a North American–style diet. (You won't, for example, need to eat rice and pickles for breakfast as is the custom in Japan.) In fact, it is recommended that you not make diet changes that are simply not practical for North American tastes or make too many changes too soon. Jumping too fast into foreign territory may

---

A Note from Dr. Jonas
START SMALL

Remember, the easiest way to stick with new eating habits, especially if they involve trying new foods and recipes, is to "think small" in the beginning. Rather than change your entire diet immediately, for example, incorporate only one new health secret or recipe from this book at a time.

Just like the person who takes up running and goes full speed for miles on day one and then can barely get out of bed the next morning, making too many diet changes at once can lead to mental overload. Invariably, that will lead to quitting—and going back to the same old routine—which, of course, is exactly what you don't want to happen.

only send you scurrying for the safety of the comforting foods of home. Both menu plans feature delicious recipes from the Global Eating recipe section starting on page 147, offering just the right amount of international flair to keep you motivated.

The Global Eating Diet Guide

This global guide will help you visualize the more than thirty secrets of the world's best diets mentioned throughout this book, so you can put them into practice. The Global Eating Diet Guide encapsulates the "secrets" of the world's healthiest diets. Consider it your map to globalizing your diet—a map that can open up a world of possibilities for both health and eating happiness.

Global Eating Plan:
Seven Days of 2,000-Calorie Menus for Weight Maintenance

MENU 1

Breakfast:
  1 cup low-fat or fat-free plain yogurt
  3 T raisin-and-almond mix
  1 tsp honey
  1 tsp flax seeds
  8 oz calcium-fortified orange juice
  Coffee or tea

Lunch:
  Miso Soup with Tofu and Wakame *(see recipe, page 150)*
  Chicken with Broccoli *(see recipe, page 169)*
  1 cup steamed brown or white rice
  1 cup fresh pineapple chunks
  Green tea

Dinner:
  Scandinavian Pork Chops in Applesauce *(see recipe, page 225)*
  1 cup wild rice
  1 cup sautéed spinach (made with 1 tsp olive oil and garlic to taste)
  Walnut Cake with Cinnamon Syrup *(see recipe, page 233)*
  Chamomile tea

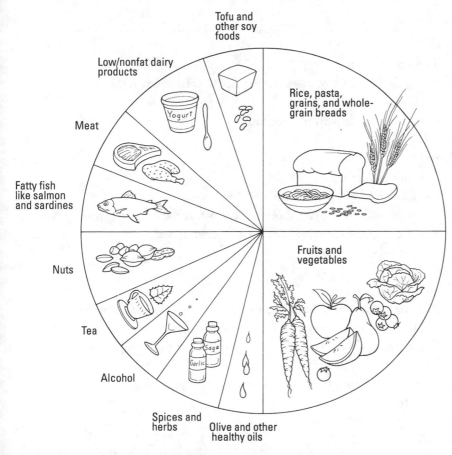

Global Guidelines:

Rice, pasta, grains, and whole-grain breads: Make these the cornerstone of your diet.

Fruits and vegetables: Strive for variety; be adventurous; serve fruit for dessert.

Olive and other healthy oils: Substitute for saturated fat, but still use sparingly.

Spices and herbs: Don't forget flavor!

Alcohol: Go ahead, but call it quits at 1–2 glasses a day.

Tea: Substitute for coffee and soda when possible.

Nuts: Don't be afraid to add them to your repertoire.

Fatty fish like salmon and sardines: Strive for 1–2 fish meals a week.

Meat: Treat like a condiment.

Low/nonfat dairy products: Make yogurt and milk everyday foods.

Tofu and other soy foods: Get more of these however you can.

Global Eating Diet Guide

MENU 2

Breakfast:

 1 cup bran flakes
 ¾ cup fat-free milk or calcium-fortified 1 percent soy milk
 1 banana
 Caffè latte (made with fat-free milk)

Lunch:

 1 ½ cups lentil soup
 1 small whole-wheat roll with 2 oz low-fat cheese
 1 cup mixed-vegetable crudité (e.g., carrots, radishes, celery, snow peas)
 8 oz fresh lemonade mixed with 8 oz sparkling water
 1 cup raspberry sorbet

Dinner:

 Arugula, Endive, and Tomato Salad with **Classic French Vinaigrette Dressing** *(see recipe, page 151)*
 Coriander-Crusted Tuna with Parsley Dressing *(see recipe, page 204)*
 1 cup herbed couscous
 1 cup fresh strawberries with ½ cup low-fat vanilla yogurt
 Mint tea

MENU 3

Breakfast:

 ½ whole-wheat bagel with 1 tsp butter or tofu spread (optional)
 2 egg whites and 1 whole egg (prepared with 1 tsp oil or butter)
 8 oz calcium-fortified orange juice
 ½ mango, sliced
 Green tea

Lunch:

 Zuppa di Finocchio *(see recipe, page 162)*
 2 slices whole-wheat bread
 Tuna salad made with:
  3 oz canned chunk light tuna, drained
  ½ cup chopped vegetables (e.g., carrots, celery, and broccoli)
  1 tsp olive oil (or 1 tsp low-fat dressing)
  balsamic vinegar or lemon juice

1 slice watermelon
Iced ginger tea sweetened with honey

Dinner:

Tsatsíki Sauce with Pita Bread *(see recipe, page 154)*
Mediterranean Roast Leg of Lamb *(see recipe, page 223)*
1 cup steamed escarole with fresh lemon juice
Assorted dried fruit (e.g., dates, figs, and apricots)
Sparkling water

MENU 4

Breakfast:

Fruit smoothie (mix in blender until smooth) made with:
    1 cup fresh or frozen blueberries (or any seasonal berry)
    ½ cup 1 percent vanilla calcium-fortified soy milk
    ½ cup low-fat vanilla yogurt
    3 ice cubes
1 small low-fat whole-grain muffin with 2 T almond or peanut butter
Green tea

Lunch:

Classic Greek Salad *(see recipe, page 155)*
1 whole-wheat pita
Dolmádas *(see recipe, page 152)*
1 banana
Iced peppermint tea with honey

Dinner:

Eggplant Szechuan-Style *(see recipe, page 184)*
Shrimp with Lobster Sauce *(see recipe, page 198)*
1 cup steamed brown or white rice
Citrus Berry Parfait *(see recipe, page 231)*
Sparkling water with lemon

MENU 5

Breakfast:

1 cup mixed-fruit salad (kiwifruit, grapes, berries)
½ pumpernickel bagel or whole-wheat baguette

2 T natural peanut butter

Tea or coffee

Lunch:

Scandinavian Fish Soup *(see recipe, page 214)*

1 cup tossed salad made with:

   dark green leafy vegetables

   tomatoes

   peppers

   carrots

   ½ cup chickpeas or pinto beans

1 T vinaigrette

3 gingersnaps or 2 fig cookies

Lemon-lime sparkling water

Dinner:

Tofu-Basil Pasta Sauce on Fettucine *(see recipe, page 185)*

Goat Cheese and Black Olive Timbales with Baby Greens *(see recipe, page 192)*

1 cup low-fat or fat-free frozen yogurt

½ cup raspberries

Chamomile tea

MENU 6

Breakfast:

Smoked Salmon Omelette with Potatoes *(see recipe, page 215)*

2 slices cantaloupe or honeydew melon

Orange spritz (4 oz calcium-fortified orange juice and 4 oz sparkling water)

Black tea

Lunch:

2 cups tossed spinach-and-mushroom salad made with:

   fresh spinach leaves

   scallions

   sliced mushrooms

   cherry tomatoes

8 black olives
1 oz feta cheese
2 T vinaigrette
1 baguette or 2 whole-grain crispbread
½ cup lemon ice
Sparkling water

Dinner:
Sautéed Chicken Breasts with Roasted Garlic Sauce *(see recipe, page 176)*
1 medium baked potato with ½ cup plain yogurt and sprinkle of chopped
    chives
Asparagus spears with 1 tsp olive oil
Orange Poppy-Seed Biscotti *(see recipe, page 232)*
1 cup vanilla low-fat frozen yogurt
Sparkling water

MENU 7

Breakfast:
1 cup oatmeal
¼ cup raisins
3 T wheat germ
1 T maple syrup
½ pink grapefruit
Coffee or tea

Lunch:
Mediterranean Tabouleh Salad *(see recipe, page 191)*
1 oz low-fat cheese
2 whole-wheat crispbread
3 oz grilled salmon or tuna (prepared with 1 tsp olive or canola oil)
1 cup steamed broccoli with lemon pepper
1 apple
Mint tea with honey

Dinner:
Curry Corn Bisque *(see recipe, page 149)*
Ginger Pork *(see recipe, page 218)*

1 cup brown rice (prepared with 1 tsp olive oil and chopped scallions)
Angel food cake with 1 T slivered almonds and 2 T raspberry sauce
Sparkling water

Global Eating Plan: Seven Days of 1,500 Calorie Menus for Weight Loss

MENU 1

Breakfast:

1 cup whole-wheat cereal
¾ cup fat-free or calcium-fortified 1 percent soy milk
½ cup sliced strawberries
Caffè latte or black tea

Lunch:

Egg Drop Soup with Tomato *(see recipe, page 148)*
Stir-Fried Tofu with Chicken and Vegetables *(see recipe, page 173)*
½ cup steamed white or brown rice
4 gingersnaps and 1 cup fat-free milk
Sparkling water

Dinner:

Chicken Yassa served with rice *(see recipe, page 180)*
1 cup steamed zucchini with lemon pepper
1 cup tropical fruit salad (kiwifruit, papaya, mango, banana) with 1T low-
   fat whipped topping
Sparkling water

MENU 2

Breakfast:

1 cup nonfat vanilla yogurt
½ cup fresh blueberries
1 tsp flax seeds
Tea or coffee

Lunch:

1 small baked, stuffed sweet potato with:

½ cup chopped steamed broccoli
2 oz melted low-fat cheese
Greek Cabbage Salad *(see recipe, page 159)*
1 orange
Water with lime

Dinner:
Grilled Salmon with Sesame Teriyaki Glaze *(see recipe, page 199)*
½ cup sautéed kale (prepared with 1 tsp olive oil and garlic to taste)
½ cup herbed couscous
Sorbetto al Cioccolato *(see recipe, page 235)*
Ginger tea

MENU 3

Breakfast:
½ whole-wheat bagel
2 T natural peanut butter
1 small tangerine
Coffee or tea

Lunch:
Hot-and-Sour Soup *(see recipe, page 147)*
Sautéed Chicken Breasts with Roasted Garlic Sauce *(see recipe, page 176)*
½ cup steamed brown or white rice
15 red grapes

Dinner:
1 cup cooked pasta with:
    1 cup mixed sautéed vegetables (broccoli, red pepper, mushrooms),
    prepared with 1 tsp olive or canola oil and 1 clove chopped garlic
1 T grated cheese
1 cup tossed mesclun salad
1 T vinaigrette
1 cup peach sorbet

MENU 4

Breakfast:
Smoked Salmon Omelette with Potatoes *(see recipe, page 215)*

1 slice honeydew melon
Green tea

Lunch:

2 cups mixed dark greens salad
½ cup chickpeas or pinto beans
1 T vinaigrette
Finnish Rye Bread *(see recipe, page 229)*
Sparkling water

Dinner:

1 cup hearty minestrone soup with grated Parmesan
Pauppiette **of Sea Bass with Tapenade and** *Sauce Provençale* **in Thin Potato Crust** *(see recipe, page 207)*
½ cup seasoned green beans (prepared with 1 tsp olive or canola oil)
Sorbetto di Limone e Basilico *(see recipe, page 234)*
Peppermint tea

MENU 5

Breakfast:

¾ cup Cheerios (or other oat cereal) and ¼ cup All-Bran cereal
¾ cup fat-free milk or calcium-fortified 1 percent soy milk
1 small banana
Green tea

Lunch:

3 oz roasted turkey or chicken in 1 small whole-wheat pita with tomato, onion, peppers, and 1 tsp mustard or low-fat mayonnaise
Sliced kiwifruit
Sparkling water with lime

Dinner:

Swedish Beef Patties with Onions *(see recipe, page 226)*
1 cup sautéed brussels sprouts (prepared with citrus juices and garlic)
1 small boiled potato
Walnut Cake with Cinnamon Syrup *(see recipe, page 233)*
Herbal tea

MENU 6

Breakfast:

    1 cup calcium-fortified fat-free or 1 percent vanilla soy milk

    Pulla *(Finnish Cardamom-Flavored Coffeebraid) (see recipe, page 228)*

    ½ cup mixed tropical fruit (mango, banana, kiwifruit, etc.)

    Coffee or tea

Lunch:

    Swedish Shrimp Salad *(see recipe, page 208)*

    1 slice whole-wheat toast

    Chamomile tea w/honey

Dinner:

    Seafood Soup with Rouille *(see recipe, page 206)*

    1½ cups mixed-greens salad with tomato, carrot ribbons, and scallions,
        and 1 T **Classic French Vinaigrette Dressing** *(see recipe, page 151)*

    Baked apple with 1 T chopped pecans

    Sparkling water

MENU 7

Breakfast:

    1 cup fat-free plain yogurt

    6 almonds or 3 Brazil nuts

    1 cup cubed cantaloupe or ¼ cup dried apricots

    1 T honey

    Black tea

Lunch:

    Mediterranean Artichoke Hearts and White Bean Stew *(see recipe,*
        page 189)

    1 small whole-wheat pita with 2 T hummus

    ½ cup low-fat frozen yogurt

    Iced tea

Dinner:

    Eggplant and Green Pepper Stir-Fry with Miso Sauce *(see recipe,*
        page 186)

Shrimp with Mixed Vegetables *(see recipe, page 202)*
½ cup steamed brown or white rice
1 cup chilled mandarin orange and pineapple salad
Sparkling water

Suggested Substitutions for Variety

The following ground rules are especially important if you plan to follow either the 1,500- or 2,000-calorie Global Eating Plan for more than a week.

- **Calorie counts:** The calorie counts are roughly the same for each breakfast, lunch, and dinner, so if you don't like one of the meals and want to replace it with one from another day—or would like to repeat a meal two days in a row—that's fine. Switching one breakfast, lunch, or dinner for another won't affect how much weight you lose, if weight loss is your goal.

- **Oils and fats:** Feel free to substitute an *equal amount* of most fats in many of these meal plans. For example, for added flavor 1 tsp of sesame oil can be used instead of 1 tsp canola oil; 1 T butter can replace 1 T olive oil. (For peanut butter, use 2 tsp for each 1 tsp of margarine or butter.) Keep in mind, however, that canola and olive oils are the preferred fats since they are highest in monounsaturated fat and lowest in saturated fat.

- **Vegetables:** Any (nonstarch) vegetable can be substituted to fit your tastes; for example, artichokes, asparagus, green beans, beets, broccoli, brussels sprouts, cabbage, carrots, cauliflower, celery, cucumber, eggplant, greens (collard, kale, mustard, turnip), kohlrabi, mushrooms, okra, peppers, radishes, salad greens, spinach, summer squash, tomatoes, watercress, zucchini. Remember, the more variety and the darker the color, the better.

- **Fruits:** Any equal amount of a compatible fruit can replace what is listed in the menus. For example, if a recipe calls for a fresh citrus fruit, you can choose from oranges, tangerines, mandarin oranges, and grapefruit. If fresh fruit isn't available, go ahead and use canned or frozen (without added sugar). When berries are listed in the menu, you can choose from any in season: strawberries, raspberries, blueberries, blackberries, cranberries.

- **Breads:** For variety, try English muffins, pita pockets, tortillas, or 100 percent whole-grain rolls.

- **Global recipes:** For variety and taste preference, any global recipe with approximately the same amount of calories and fat can be substituted in these meal plans. To keep the carbohydrate, protein, and fats balanced, however, try to choose a recipe from the same nutrient category. For example, feel free to substitute any suggested chicken recipe for another chicken or fish recipe, any soup recipe for another soup recipe, and so on. The calories and fat in the recipes you substitute just need to be roughly the same as the recipe originally suggested.

- Drink as much water, seltzer, or herbal tea as you like, but limit your intake of caffeinated beverages such as coffee, tea, or diet cola to two or three servings a day.

9

Global Eating Ground Rules for Navigating Your Diet in a New Direction

While the 1,500- and 2,000-calorie eating plans make it convenient for you to begin incorporating more trailblazing ways of eating to reduce your risk of disease, you don't need to follow specific menu plans to master the art of Global Eating. To take your diet in a healthier direction, just keep the following basic global guidelines in mind (which are conveniently mined from the extensive list of global secrets mentioned throughout this book) when you're shopping, chopping, cooking, and dining.

- **Get picky.** When giving your diet the power of produce (Global Eating Secret #8—China), take note also from the French and the people of the Mediterranean. For best flavor and highest nutritional value, be particular. It's easier to learn to love fruits and vegetables if what you're buying is at its peak flavor and intensity. How do you know you're buying the best produce for the buck? "Squeeze it," any Sicilian or French shopper is likely to advise you. "If it's too hard, it's not ripe enough. If it's too soft, it's too ripe." (After a while, "the feel test" becomes almost innate.) Also, get nosy. With certain fruits such as peaches and melons, a strong scent means they're appropriately ripening. (Don't waste your time, however, thumping or shaking a melon in the produce aisle like it's a percussion instrument. A hollow echo is no indication of ripeness.) Also, although there's no need to limit yourself to what's in season since a variety of fruits and vegetables are available year-round throughout North America, for maximum enjoyment and peak flavor, take advantage of the fresh-picked jewels each season has to offer. Here's a quick hit list by season:

1 **Spring:** Asparagus, artichokes, carrots, leeks, lettuce, new potatoes, peas, radishes, rhubarb, scallions, spinach, and strawberries.

2 **Summer:** Apricots, bell peppers, blackberries, blueberries, cantaloupe, cherries, cucumbers, eggplant, fresh herbs, grapes, green beans, honeydew, hot peppers, nectarines, okra, peaches, peppers, plums, raspberries, scallions, summer squash, strawberries, sweet corn, tomatoes, watermelon, and zucchini.

3 **Fall:** Apples, beets, broccoli, brussels sprouts, cabbage, cauliflower, collard greens, cranberries, endive, grapes, kale, pears, persimmons, pineapple, pumpkin, spinach, winter squash, and sweet potatoes.

4 **Winter:** Beets, cabbage, carrots, citrus fruit, daikon radishes, onions, rutabagas, turnips, and winter squash.

- **Be a risk taker.** The produce aisle is a good place to begin sampling the growing variety of exotic fruits, vegetables, and beans now available at many supermarkets across North America (right in line with Global Eating Secret #18: Savor Variety). Expanding your horizons can help fight a ho-hum attitude about produce that can creep into your repertoire. (You know this is happening to you when you have thoughts such as *Broccoli again?*) As discussed, a varied diet, especially in the fruit and vegetable category, can also provide extra health insurance against diseases such as cancer, because each fruit or vegetable offers its own profile of substances and nutrients that tend to work as a team to protect against disease. The table below reviews just some of the "foreign" fruits, vegetables, and beans mentioned throughout this book and tells you how to use them and what nutrients they provide.

Be on the Lookout for This Produce

PRODUCE AND HOMELAND	LOOKS LIKE	TASTES	GOOD SOURCE OF	PREPARATION
Bok choy (China)	Wide-stalked celery with dark green leaves	Mild	Beta-carotene and vitamin C	Use raw in salads; toss stems and hearts in a stir-fry.

Daikon radish (Japan)	An overgrown white carrot	Sweet, fresh	Vitamin C	Use raw in salads; shred as a garnish; toss in a stir-fry.
Cassava (Africa)	A large brown foot-long potato covered with hairy bark	Nutlike	Fiber	Peel and cook like potatoes; serve with a spicy sauce.
Fava (broad) beans (the Mediterranean)	Large lima beans	Pealike	Fiber, protein, iron, and folate	Blanch and remove the thick skins before cooking. Combine peeled beans with herbs, and boil in water until tender. Serve in salads or as a side dish; toss into soups.
Broccoli raab (the Mediterranean)	Leafy, thin, dark green broccoli stalks with tiny, tight cluster buds	Pungent, slightly bitter	Beta-carotene and vitamin C	Chop up and steam or sauté; toss raw into salads and soups.
Shiitake mushrooms (Japan)	Large brown cap with skinny white stem	Full-bodied and chewy	Niacin and riboflavin (B vitamins), potassium, and iron	Sauté, broil, or bake; use in stir-fries and sauces.
Fresh ginger (China)	Knobby tan-colored root	Sweet, pungent	No identifiable nutrient properties— yet; but a smart way to add flavor to low-fat foods	Grated or chopped, ginger can be used in stir-fries, marinades, breads, salads, soups, and stews.
Curly or Italian parsley (the Mediterranean)	Curly green leaves or flat, pointed leaves	Mild or pungent	Excellent source of anti-oxidant vitamin C and beta-carotene	Use in salads, soups, stews, dips, and both vegetable and meat dishes.

PRODUCE AND HOMELAND	LOOKS LIKE	TASTES	GOOD SOURCE OF	PREPARATION
Mustard greens (China)	A daintier rendition of kale with ruffled, grass-green leaves	Peppery	Superb source of vitamin A	Serve as an accompaniment or toss into soups, stews, and casseroles.
Papaya (a sought-after newcomer in Scandinavia)	An over-grown light-bulb with creamy yellow skin	Sweet and refreshing	Great source of vitamin C	Serve solo for dessert.
Mango (ditto)	An odd-shaped ball with red-orange skin	A cross between a peach and a pineapple	Rich in beta-carotene	Ditto
Kiwifruit (ditto)	A brown, hairy egg with a fleshy chartreuse interior	A cross between a strawberry and a melon	Tops in vitamin C	Toss in fruit salads or eat on its own as a treat.
Napa cabbage (China)	Long heads of light-green lettuce with crinkly, thick leaves	Mild	Calcium and vitamin A	Sauté or toss into a stir-fry.

- **Make traditional American side dishes your entrée.** Besides more fruits and vegetables, eating more low-fat complex carbohydrates is one of the most important diet secrets from foreign lands to consider introducing into your diet. In many of the countries covered in this book meat is traditionally consumed in garnish proportions to merely flavor the rest of the meal. Or, as in the Mediterranean, it's consumed in greater quantities, but not every day. Meanwhile, whole grains like rice and whole-grain breads (Global Eating Secret #24), beans and lentils (Global Eating Secret #5), as well as vegetables and fruits fill in the gaps.

  Giving up the notion that meals revolve around meat may be the toughest adjustment you will have to make to globalize your eating habits. Many of us, after all, were raised on meat-centered meals. But nonetheless, try to be a meat minimalist (Global Eating Secret #10), using meat as simply a way to flavor vegetables and grains.

On days when you just want to eat the good, old-fashioned, American way, however, try to put the brakes on. Make your serving of meat no larger than a floppy disk. Meanwhile, prepare a bounty of veggies—say, a salad, green beans, and a baked potato—to give you plenty of great stuff to help you fill up. Ideally, strive to make vegetables at least half your plate.

Your Primer to Selecting the Leanest Meats

When you must have meat, it pays not only to keep your servings small-ish but to make wiser choices at the meat counter. If you search hard enough, you can find low-fat options. With this in mind, here's a primer to navigating the meat counter and choosing the skinniest cuts.

- **Beef.** The skinniest cuts generally have "loin" or "round" in the name. A 3-ounce serving of eye of round, for example, has roughly 140 calories and 4 grams of fat—half the fat and calories as the same size serving of a heftier option like spare ribs. Other low-fat cuts of beef to look for at the meat counter include top round, round tip, eye of round, sirloin, top loin, and tenderloin.

- **Ground Beef.** Critics would argue that there's no such thing as low-fat ground beef, because even the lowest fat choices available have about 10 grams of fat per 3-ounce serving. But some ground beef is leaner than others. To choose the skinniest options, keep these hints in mind: Aim for packages labeled at least "90 percent lean," which indicates the lean-to-fat ratio of 90 percent meat to 10 percent fat. The maximum proportion of leanness is "95 percent lean"—an even better option if it's available in your supermarket. The original cut from which the ground beef came will also clue you in. Search for "ground round," the leanest ground beef in the meat department, or for "ground sirloin." A drawback: They are usually the most expensive option. Steer clear of "ground chuck" or "regular ground beef," which is generally 70 percent lean and 30 percent fat.

- **Pork, Lamb, and Veal.** Skinny cuts of pork, veal, or lamb are labeled "loin" or "leg." A 3-ounce serving of pork tenderloin, for example, has roughly 140 calories and 4 grams of fat, compared to a pork chop that weighs in at an average of 190 calories and 8 grams of fat. Other lean choices include pork boneless top loin chops and center loin chops; lamb loin chops or legs; veal cutlets or veal chops.

- **Chicken and Turkey.** Stick to white meat, yet watch out for the wing. It's often considered white, yet it's fattier than the drumstick without the skin. Ounce per ounce, dark chicken meat can be higher in fat than beef round steak or sirloin. And when it comes to ground chicken or turkey, look for those that specify ground "breast meat." Labels that simply state "ground turkey" or "ground chicken" mean that you're buying meat plus skin, which has ten times more fat than the skinless version. If ground breast meat isn't available, ask the butcher to grind up turkey or chicken breasts without the skin. Use as you would ground beef.

What about Grade?

The USDA grades of beef, lamb, and veal—Prime, Choice, and Select—are determined by the amount of integral fat, or "marbling," contained in a piece of meat. Thus they're a key to leanness. (Pork is not on a grading system.) But don't let the grade bog you down. Here's why:

Meat labeled Prime is nearly 10 percent fat and considered the most succulent option. But not to worry about temptation at home—prime meat is usually offered only in specialty food markets and restaurants. Meat graded Choice (about 7 percent fat) and Select (the leanest grade at 6 percent fat) are probably the two options you'll have.

The difference between a 3-ounce serving of Select and a 3-ounce piece of Choice meat amounts to only about 2 grams of fat. But if this small fat difference is important to you, seek out Select. If it's not available at your supermarket, ask the butcher to order it. Otherwise, buy Choice meat and trim the fat before cooking.

- **Drink tea instead of coffee or soda** (*Global Eating Secret #12*). As mentioned in the chapter on China, green tea or black teas such as Earl

Grey, English breakfast, and regular Lipton contain polyphenols, powerful antioxidants that research shows may help reduce your risk of heart disease and certain cancers. Tea is an important beverage in the global diet. If caffeine is a worry, simply switch to decaf. Keep in mind, however, that herbal tea doesn't wield the same disease-fighting power because it doesn't come from tea leaves.

- **Make arrangements at mealtime** (*Global Eating Secret #20*). When it comes to global eating, appearance counts, too. To make low-fat, lower-calorie foods more tempting and satisfying, take note from the Japanese, who are fond of manipulating the appearance of their meals as carefully as a bonsai tree. Is there a balance of form, color, and texture? Do your meals look appetizing? For the greatest gratification per calorie, the Japanese would politely remind you to pay attention to how food is presented on your plate.

- **Include more fish.** Start with at least one fish meal a week (Global Eating Secret #21), and go from there. Fatty fish such as salmon, bluefish, sardines, herring, and mackerel are prevalent in both the Japanese and the Nordic diets. Rich in heart-healthy and brain-nourishing omega-3 fatty acids and in protein, fish is perhaps one of the world's most underrated foods. Do yourself a favor and work it into your diet as often as you can. For an extra dose of omega-3 fatty acids (Global Eating Secret #2), also consider adding walnuts, canola oil, flaxseeds and flaxseed oil, as well as leafy green vegetables to your routine.

- **Try tofu, tempeh, and other soy foods.** As mentioned in Global Eating Secret #22, soy foods are a good, lower-fat substitute for meat on occasion. To save more than half the calories and fat, however, be sure to choose light tofu over regular versions. For tofu ideas, see the Global Vegetarian recipes in chapter 10.

- **Switch to "healthy" fats** (*Global Eating Secret #12*). Monounsaturated fats such as olive and canola oils have been shown to change the fat chemistry of the blood to reduce the risk of heart disease and cancer—a good reason to substitute them for the butter, margarine, and corn oil in your diet whenever possible. When sautéing or stir-frying, remember to use just enough olive or canola oil to barely coat the bottom of the pan, since all oils—heart-healthy or not—contain roughly 120 calories per tablespoon. Also, steer clear of processed foods made with palm, palm kernel, or coconut oils (wisdom gleaned from western Africa). These tropical oils are akin to saturated fat and thus just as unhealthy as if they were laden with butter.

- **If you drink, remember—a little goes a long way** *(Global Eating Secret #15)*. Studies show that a little alcohol in your diet can be healthy for your heart, but to avoid increasing your risk of other conditions, set your limit at no more than one glass a day (women) or two glasses a day (men). One glass equals 12 ounces of beer, 4 to 5 ounces of wine, or 1.5 ounces of 80-proof liquor. Cheers! Or as they say in France, "To your health!"

- **Fiber up your diet with beans and whole-grain breads and cereal** *(Global Eating Secrets #5 and #24)*. Fiber may be an effective cancer fighter by speeding waste through the digestive tract; it also helps lower blood cholesterol and blood pressure and slows the breakdown of carbohydrates, which may be beneficial for people with Type 2 diabetes. Moreover, a high-fiber diet may help you keep your weight in check by helping you absorb fewer calories.

- **Learn to love low-fat and fat-free dairy foods** *(Global Eating Secret #25)*. North Americans don't have to become as dairy crazed as the Scandinavians, but we could stand to pay more attention to the low-fat and fat-free options in this food group. The calcium as well as the complete package of nutrients contained in dairy products may not only help prevent bone-thinning osteoporosis in both men and women but also help fight high blood pressure, colon cancer, and perhaps even breast cancer, as well as help combat symptoms of PMS such as irritability, anxiety, and mood swings.

- **Jazz up meals** *(Global Eating Secrets #4 and #29)*. Make herbs, spices, and nonfat sauces your best friends. They tantalize your tongue, giving you a heightened sense of satisfaction with each bite. With such good company, who needs butter, margarine, or corn oil (the traditional North American though less than healthy way to flavor meals)? Experiment when you're cooking with no-fat flavor enhancers such as parsley and rosemary (both of which offer antioxidants), garlic and vinegars (red, white, and balsamic), Dijon mustard, low-sodium soy sauce (in moderation), Chinese Five-Spice Powder, onions, cayenne, and other hot peppers, as well as *herbes de Provence* (a classic southern France combination of basil, fennel seed, lavender, marjoram, rosemary, sage, summer savory, and thyme). Look for it on supermarket shelves and in specialty stores.

Exercising for Global Health

To stay healthy for the long haul, your diet is only one part of the equation. As you probably know, an active lifestyle invigorates the heart, enabling it to pump more blood with each beat. Regular exercise can lower your total cholesterol and LDL (bad) cholesterol, and raise HDL (good) cholesterol. It also reduces blood pressure and helps build or at least preserve muscle mass, something that otherwise gradually diminishes as you get older. Weight-bearing activities like walking also help strengthen bones to prevent osteoporosis. Exercise also helps to boost mood and is the single activity most clearly associated with long-term weight maintenance.

Finding the time for exercise in your life means making exercise a priority and scheduling it in regularly. To get started, start slow. Schedule three ten-minute sessions a week at a time that's convenient for you. After you've done that for two weeks or so, then go to twenty minutes three times a week, and so on. In the beginning, it doesn't matter how long you exercise or how hard you work, just that you're exercising regularly. This is one of the most effective ways to get in shape "the North American way."

If a formal exercise program isn't for you, know that you can still do your body good by getting bouts of exercise throughout your day. In fact, this is how the citizens of many of the countries mentioned in this book prefer to exercise. Besides diet, another clue to the leanness and "heartiness" of the French, for example, are their exercise habits. Yes, you'll find health clubs in France, especially in the major cities like Paris, where racquetball sessions and aerobic classes convene daily. But there are not as many as you see in North America. Customarily, sweating up a storm at a health club is not the way the French prefer to strut their stuff. They don't consider working out for an hour on the weight machine *civilized*. Instead, many leave their cars at home (after all, there's often no place to park at work or at the market), and set out *à pied* (on foot). "No one climbs more steps than Métro-taking Parisians, nor carries heavier loads than the French do coming home from the market," writes Susan Hermann Loomis. For fun, the French are apt to hit a section of the 19,000 miles of *Grandes Randonnées* (long-distance tracks) throughout France's national park system.

Besides walking and taking the stairs, gardening is also big in France, for those who have the space. So is doing your own dishes, since many homes and apartments don't have dishwashers. It's also common in France to do your own housework, which can burn an average of 420 calories an hour if you scrub that tile and vacuum vigorously. Also, many city apartments are exquisite multifloor walk-ups; elevators are often reserved for only the newest buildings, limited though they are. And even if you're lucky enough to live in an elevator building in France, it's considered bad manners to take the elevator down unless you're handicapped or loaded with the baggage you're taking on a trip. No matter where you live in France, you're destined to use the stairclimber and the treadmill that nature and urban architecture graciously and generously offers.

Similarly, in Beijing, a city of more than 13 million, each day a sea of sturdy bicycles dominates the streets, competing with cars for road space. Bicycles outnumber the 1.2 million cars there by more than five to one. And it seems everybody rides—middle-aged lab technicians, restaurateurs, librarians—not just bicycle messengers. Many people think nothing of riding 5 miles or more to work, something to keep in mind the next time you hesitate to take the stairs at your office or get off the bus several stops early to foot it the rest of the way.

While such low-key activities as weeding may not compete with an hour workout at the gym, every little bit of movement can incinerate calories. Moderately intense activities such as walking at a brisk pace or taking the dog for a hike after dinner won't help you build up your muscles or train for a sport, but studies show that *activating* your day can help you burn more calories to achieve and maintain a healthy weight and boost your overall fitness level. An extra fifteen minutes of brisk walking a day, for example, can burn an average of 575 calories a week, which can add up to an 8-pound weight loss over a year's time. In fact, short bouts of exercise throughout your day can help reduce your risk of cardiovascular disease and osteoporosis as well as improve your mood and your balance, coordination, and agility.

Aside from a regular exercise program, you have dozens of opportunities each day to become more active—ways that don't involve any special equipment or a trip to the gym. Here are eight to help get you started.

Pace when you're talking on the phone instead of staying put. Though not a significant calorie-burner, getting up often out of your chair throughout the day can help boost your circulation.

If you have a fireplace or wood-burning stove, chop your own wood. It's laborious, but just think of the calorie burn: an average of 450 calories in fifteen minutes (that's roughly the number of calories in a McDonald's Grilled Chicken Deluxe). Stack the firewood, and you'll expend an additional 18 calories per minute.

Deliver memos in person. Resist the urge to have your assistant do it, send them via e-mail, or fax them from floor to floor. Consider these excursions exercise breaks.

Clean your house vigorously. Cleaning floors with a flourish, vacuuming carpets with a vengeance, washing windows and scrubbing tile with style can add up to hundreds of "reps," and a calorie burn of roughly 420 calories an hour.

Do your own yard work and gardening. You'll think of weeds as your friends when you consider that hoeing burns roughly 360 calories per hour, akin to playing badminton. Likewise, cutting your lawn with a push mower is on the same calorie par as playing tennis (420 calories per hour). And at 500 calories per hour, trimming trees is equivalent to swimming a slow crawl.

Sideline your electric mixer or food processor. For an upper-body workout, beat, whip, and chop ingredients by hand, and put some muscle into it. Kneading bread dough is also great exercise for your biceps, forearms, and hands. To work dough for as long as the recipe recommends (that's usually ten minutes, which can feel much longer), however, set a timer, put on your favorite CD or radio station, and knead to the beat.

Turn lunchtime into an adventure. Instead of going to the cafeteria or out to eat at the same place around the corner, make a point of discovering new restaurants at least five blocks from your workplace. There's nothing like having a culinary destination to put a spring in your step.

Think of flights in terms of calories. To motivate yourself to take the stairs instead of the elevator or escalator, keep in mind that each flight you ascend burns roughly 10 calories. That doesn't sound like much, but taking ten flights a day over the course of a year can add up to a 10-pound weight loss.

Recipes from the Global Kitchen

Leave a little room in your stomach. Try to stay lean for the sake of health and motivation. The mind grows sluggish on too much rich food and fine wine.

—Ancient Tao principle

If you're interested in changing your diet so that it reflects the culinary wisdom of the countries discussed in this book, what better place to start than in your own kitchen. To help you jump-start your efforts, a host of cooking professionals have contributed recipes that can help you bring home the flavors and the secrets of healthy eating from Japan, China, France, the Mediterranean, Scandinavia, and Africa.

By making these recipes part of your everyday repertoire, you'll automatically put into practice many Global Eating principles—such as eating plenty of fruits and vegetables; reducing animal products by eating tofu and grains and without sacrificing flavor; eating more fish; and introducing healthy fats like olive oil into your diet. While some recipes call for mainstream ingredients, others require items you can usually find in your supermarket's international section or at specialty markets.

Most of the recipes that follow are low in fat. Some, however, such as the traditional recipes from the Mediterranean, make more liberal use of olive oil. When preparing these recipes, be sure to balance your fat and calories at subsequent meals. Remember, to stick to a low-fat diet—the Global Eating Secret the Chinese and Japanese, especially, have been putting into practice for centuries—try to keep your total fat intake at no more than 30 percent of total calories *over the course of a week,* not to any one food. As we've learned from the people of the Mediterranean and especially the French, there truly is room in your diet for a variety of foods—even higher-fat ones—occasionally. *Bon appétit!*

The Global Eating Pantry

With a well-stocked pantry and freezer, you'll have the basics for countless Global Eating meals within arm's reach. Here's a general list of global ingredients to have on hand. With a packed global pantry, you'll be in and out of the supermarket in record time. Your grocery list will need to include only the staples you're low on, plus the fresh ingredients you need each week to prepare the global recipes you've chosen.

Broths:	nonfat chicken broth
Vegetables with a lengthy shelf life:	grape leaves (preserved in jar)
	onions
	shallots
Freezer meats and seafood:	chicken
	ground pork or chicken
	lean ground beef
	leg of lamb
	pork loin
	salmon fillets
	sea bass
	shrimp
	sirloin beef
	smoked salmon
	swordfish
Nuts and dried fruits:	currants
	peanuts
	pine nuts (store in freezer so they don't spoil)
	sliced almonds
Condiments, sauces, and oils:	bamboo shoots
	canola oil
	capers
	Chinese black vinegar*
	dashi*
	Dijon mustard
	dried black mushrooms*
	dried lily flower buds*
	dried tree ears*
	dry white wine

fish sauce*
green olives
hoisin sauce*
honey
hot bean paste*
Kalamata olives
ketchup
lemon juice
low-sodium soy sauce
mirin (available at liquor stores)
miso*
olive oil
oyster sauce*
pickled ginger*
red wine vinegar
rice wine
sake
sesame oil
sweet bean sauce*
water chestnuts
Worcestershire sauce

Herbs, spices, and other flavor makers:

bay leaves
black olives
cardamom seeds
cayenne pepper
chili paste
Chinese Five-Spice Powder
cinnamon
coriander seeds
cumin (both ground and seeds)
curry powder
dried red chilies
garlic
ginger root
herbes de Provence
instant coffee
kosher salt
orange extract
oregano
paprika
poppy seeds

	rosemary
	saffron
	thyme
	vanilla
	wasabi powder*
	white pepper
Dry and canned goods:	anchovies
	bean thread noodles*
	bread crumbs
	brown sugar
	cellophane noodles*
	chickpeas (garbanzo beans)
	cocoa powder
	cornstarch
	dried lo mein noodles*
	farina
	fettuccine
	fish stock
	flour
	macaroni shells
	nori*
	pickled beets
	raisins
	salt
	soba noodles*
	sugar
	tabouleh (bulgur wheat)
	unflavored gelatin
	white or brown rice
	whole-grain rye flour (available at health food stores)
	whole tomatoes
	yeast

*Available at Asian or specialty markets

Hot-and-Sour Soup

—Lan Tan

Serves 6 to 8

Marinade:

1 tsp low-sodium soy sauce

1 tsp rice wine

1 tsp cornstarch

¼ lb boneless, skinless chicken breast, julienned

4 dried black mushrooms

2 T dried tree ears

¼ cup dried lily flower buds

¼ cup (1 oz) fresh bean sprouts

6 cups low-sodium or low-fat chicken broth

1 T low-sodium soy sauce

Pinch sugar

¾ cup firm, light tofu, julienned

3 T cornstarch, dissolved in 2 T water

3 T black vinegar

½ tsp white pepper

1 egg, slightly beaten

1 tsp sesame oil

chili oil to taste (optional)

2 whole scallions, finely chopped

1 In a small bowl, combine marinade ingredients. Add julienned chicken, and toss to coat. Cover with plastic wrap and refrigerate 30 minutes.

2 Soak mushrooms, tree ears, and lily flower buds in hot water in separate bowls for 20 minutes or until soft, then drain.

3 Coarsely chop mushrooms and bean sprouts.

4 Wash the tree ears carefully, then julienne into thin strips.

5 In a large pot, bring the chicken broth to a boil over medium-high heat. Add soy sauce and sugar, then add the mushrooms, tree ears, lily buds, and bean sprouts. Boil for 1 minute. Add tofu. Bring to a boil again. Stir in cornstarch mixture for 1 minute or until soup thickens.

6 Add the vinegar and white pepper. Stir well. Add the marinated chicken and beaten egg, and cook until chicken turns white, 1 to 2 minutes. Turn off heat.

7 Garnish with sesame oil, chili oil, and scallions.

Nutrition Information Per Serving	
Calories 85	Protein (g) 10
Fat (g) 2.5	Sodium (mg) 380
Fiber (g) . . . . >1	Carbohydrates (g) 8.5
	Cholesterol (mg) 30

Egg Drop Soup with Tomato

Serves 6 to 8

—*Lan Tan*

6 cups fat-free or sodium-free
   chicken broth

1 T low-sodium soy sauce

Pinch white pepper

2 (1 cup) tomatoes, diced

3 oz (½ cup) firm, light tofu,
   diced

3 T cornstarch, dissolved in ¼
   cup water

2 eggs, lightly beaten with 2 tsp
   rice wine

1 tsp sesame oil

2 T chopped scallions

1 In large pot, bring the chicken broth to a boil. Add soy sauce, white pepper, and diced tomato. Boil for about 2 minutes.

2 Add tofu gently. Stir in dissolved cornstarch, stirring continuously until soup is thickened, about 1 minute.

3 Mix in beaten egg mixture. Stir well. Turn off heat. Garnish with sesame oil and chopped scallions. Serve hot.

Nutrition Information Per Serving			
Calories 65		Protein (g) 10.5	
Fat (g) 2		Sodium (mg) 490	
Fiber (g) . . . . >1		Carbohydrates (g) 8	
		Cholesterol (mg) 45	

Curry Corn Bisque

—Anne Patterson

Serves 4

1 Heat oil in a large pot over medium heat. Add chopped onion, corn, curry powder, ginger, salt, and cayenne. Stir and cook for 10 minutes. Remove from heat.

2 Drain tofu, cut up and put into a food processor, and blend until smooth. Stop and scrape down sides of food processor bowl.

3 Add half of the corn mixture and about ½ cup of the chicken broth to bowl of food processor and blend with tofu until fairly smooth.

4 Scrape mixture from food processor into large pot of remaining corn mixture. Add all of the remaining broth. Stir and bring to a simmer. Cook 5 minutes, stirring occasionally. Season with salt to taste. Evenly distribute into four soup bowls. Garnish each with 1 tablespoon of finely sliced green onion.

1 T oil

1 ½ cups coarsely chopped onion

3 cups fresh corn or frozen corn, thawed

1 tsp curry powder

½ tsp finely grated raw peeled ginger

¼ tsp salt

⅛ tsp cayenne pepper

One 12.3-oz block extra-firm or firm silken tofu

2 cups nonfat chicken broth

¼ cup thinly sliced green onion tops

Nutrition Information Per Serving

Calories 200	Protein (g) 13
Fat (g) 6	Sodium (mg) 415
Fiber (g) 4.5	Carbohydrates (g) 30
	Cholesterol (mg) 0

Miso Soup with Tofu and Wakame

Serves 4

—*Kiyoko Konishi*

1 T wakame seaweed*

3 cups dashi (bonito stock)*

½ block (1 cup) silken tofu, cut
    into small dice

1 T red miso (fermented soybean
    paste)

scallions, thinly sliced

Available at Japanese markets

1 Soak wakame in water for 5 minutes or until reconstituted. Cut into bite-size pieces.

2 In a medium pot, bring dashi to a boil over medium-high heat. Add wakame and boil for 1 to 2 minutes. Add tofu and lower heat to simmer.

3 In a small bowl, dissolve miso with ½ cup of broth from the pot; return to the pot.

4 Just before broth boils, add scallions and turn off heat.

Nutrition Information Per Serving	
Calories 175	Protein (g) 10
Fat (g) 4	Sodium (mg) 1795
Fiber (g) 3	Carbohydrates (g) 25
	Cholesterol (mg) 2

Classic French Vinaigrette Dressing

—Lynn Kutner

Mix all ingredients except oil in a small bowl. Slowly whisk in oil to form a thick emulsion. Taste to correct for salt and pepper. Add a few more drops of oil if it tastes too sharp. Toss with greens such as arugula, butter lettuce, and/or radicchio.

Juice of half a lemon or lime

1 to 3 tsp Dijon mustard

1/8 to 1/4 tsp fresh ground pepper

1 small pressed clove of garlic (optional)

Pinch of dried herbs (such as *herbes de Provence,* basil, or oregano)

1/4 to 1/3 cup extra-virgin olive oil

Salt

Nutrition Information Per Tablespoon

Calories	45	Protein (g)	1
Fat (g)	4.5	Sodium (mg)	16
Fiber (g)	>1	Carbohydrates (g)	1
		Cholesterol (mg)	0

Dolmádas (Stuffed Grape Leaves)

Serves 6

—Amanda Cushman

¼ cup currants

1 cup dry white wine

¾ cup olive oil

6 scallions, chopped

2 T chopped parsley

¾ cup white rice

1 T dill

¼ cup toasted pine nuts

Salt and pepper

1 jar grape leaves*

3 lemons, juiced

2 cups nonfat chicken broth

Lemon wedges, for garnish

*Available at Middle Eastern and international markets.

1 Combine the currants and white wine in a bowl and set aside for 10 minutes.

2 Warm 1 T of the olive oil in a medium saucepan; sauté the scallions for 2 minutes. Add parsley, rice, dill, pine nuts, currant mixture, and salt and pepper to taste. Bring to a simmer; cover and cook until liquid is absorbed, about 10 minutes. Uncover and cool.

3 Blanch grape leaves for 30 seconds; drain, dry, and arrange shiny side down on counter. Cut out tough stems.

4 Place a teaspoon of rice filling in each, and roll like an egg roll. Place in a large oblong baking dish (not Pyrex), and arrange seam-side down, fitting together in a single layer. Sprinkle with lemon juice and olive oil. Continue stacking them on top of each other in layers, using up all the lemon and oil.

5 Preheat oven to 350°F.

6 Pour chicken broth around edges. Place a plate on top to weigh down, and cover with foil. Bake for 40 minutes or until rice is tender. Serve with lemon wedges at room temperature.

Nutrition Information Per Serving (4 dolmádas)	
Calories 205	Protein (g) 6
Fat (g) 5.5	Sodium (mg) 130
Fiber (g) 2	Carbohydrates (g) 30
	Cholesterol (mg) 0

Crostini with Chèvre and Tomato Garnish

—Amanda Cushman

Makes 15

1 Heat oven to 400°F. Brush bread lightly with 2 T olive oil, and toast in the oven until lightly browned, about 10 minutes.

2 Heat 1 T olive oil in a medium skillet and sauté the garlic, rosemary, and thyme for 1 minute. Remove from heat and transfer to a medium bowl.

3 Add cheese and mix well.

4 Spread the cheese lightly on crostini; garnish with the chopped tomatoes.

1 baguette, thinly sliced

Olive oil

4 cloves garlic, minced

1 T chopped fresh rosemary (or 2 tsp dried)

2 tsp chopped fresh thyme (or 1 tsp dried)

6 oz chèvre (goat cheese)

3 plum tomatoes, finely chopped, for garnish

Nutrition Information Per Crostini

Calories 155	Protein (g) 6	
Fat (g) 6.5	Sodium (mg) 225	
Fiber (g) 1	Carbohydrates (g) 15	
	Cholesterol (mg) 10	

Tsatsíki Sauce (Mediterranean Yogurt-Cucumber Dip) with Pita Bread

Serves 12

2 medium cucumbers, peeled
   and seeded

Salt and pepper

2 cups plain nonfat yogurt

1 to 2 T olive oil

2 cloves garlic, minced

2 T snipped chives or dill

8 pitas, cut in triangles

Olive oil

—Amanda Cushman

Tzatzíki, a refreshing yogurt sauce, can be eaten with a simple slice of pita bread, as a dip for fresh vegetables, or as a sauce for grilled vegetables, fish, lamb, or chicken. Besides its versatility, it's very low in calories.

1 Grate the cucumber and place in a sieve over a bowl for 30 minutes, refrigerated.

2 Heat oven to 400°F.

3 Combine the cucumbers, salt, pepper, yogurt, olive oil, garlic, and herbs in a small bowl and mix well. Taste for seasoning. Makes 2 cups.

4 Lay the triangles of pita on a baking sheet and drizzle with a little olive oil. Bake until golden, about 10 minutes. Serve with dip.

Nutrition Information Per Serving (2 T dip with 2 pita triangles)

Calories 115		Protein (g) 5	
Fat (g) 1		Sodium (mg) 185	
Fiber (g) 1		Carbohydrates (g) 20	
		Cholesterol (mg) 1	

Classic Greek Salad

—*Amanda Cushman*

Serves 8

1 Halve the cucumbers lengthwise; remove seeds and cut into ½-inch chunks. Sprinkle with salt, and allow to drain in a sieve for about 30 minutes, refrigerated. Then place in a salad bowl.

2 Halve onions and cut in ½-inch chunks; add to cucumber. Cut tomatoes into large chunks and add to the bowl.

3 Sprinkle the cheese on top and gently toss. Add mint, lemon juice, olive oil, olives, and salt and pepper. Toss again. Chill.

2 cucumbers

Salt

2 small red onions

4 ripe tomatoes

8 oz feta cheese, crumbled

5 T fresh mint, chopped

3 lemons, juiced

3 T olive oil

½ cup black Kalamata olives

salt and pepper

Nutrition Information Per Serving	
Calories 210	Protein (g) 6
Fat (g) 15	Sodium (mg) 410
Fiber (g) 3	Carbohydrates (g) 15
	Cholesterol (mg) 25

Greek Marinated Roasted Peppers

Serves 6

3 red peppers (or a combination
    of yellow and orange),
    roasted or grilled

4 T olive oil

1 T vinegar

1 clove garlic, minced

Salt and pepper

—Nikki Rose

In Greece, you rarely see people eating full meals with everything combined on one plate. Most things are served family-style on separate plates and everyone nibbles for hours. Typically, you'll see grilled or sautéed meats or fish and many little vegetable selections with lots of bread to dip in the various sauces. Here is a colorful cold *meze* (literally "little plate") or garnish for main courses.

1 Roast or grill peppers. *To roast,* rub peppers lightly with olive oil and roast on a baking pan in the oven at 400°F until the skin starts to brown and blister (about 1 hour). Set aside to cool. *To grill peppers,* rub them lightly with olive oil; grill on a stove burner or a grill until the skin starts to blacken and blisters. Place in a bowl and cover. Set aside to cool. If using different colored peppers, use separate bowls for each color.

2 Carefully remove the skin, seeds, and ribs from peppers and slice into ½-inch-wide strips. In most cases, there's always a problem spot where the skin won't budge—not to worry—it's edible.

3 In a bowl large enough to fit the peppers, whisk the olive oil, vinegar, and seasonings together. Add the peppers; cover and refrigerate until ready to use. Keeps for 1 week under refrigeration.

4 Serve with olives, marinated artichoke hearts, steamed asparagus, and other *meze* items.

Nutrition Information Per Serving

Calories 10	Protein (g) 6
Fat (g) . . . . >1	Sodium (mg) 0
Fiber (g) . . . . >1	Carbohydrates (g) . . . . >1
	Cholesterol (mg) 0

Roasted Beets

—Nikki Rose

Another refreshing and classic Greek *meze* dish.

1 Preheat oven to 375°F. Remove beet greens and reserve for another use. Rinse and scrub beets, and drain.

2 In a 9 × 13-inch heavy baking pan, add beets, onion, cloves, olive oil, and vinegar; toss to coat. Cover with foil, and roast until tender (about I hour). Remove from oven to cool.

3 Peel beets, and slice into quarters.

4 Sauté with a splash of vinegar; salt, and pepper to taste.

Serves 6

1 to 2 bunches of beets (allow 2 or 3 medium beets per person)

1 small red onion, sliced

2 garlic cloves, sliced

2 T olive oil

3 T red wine vinegar

Salt and pepper

Nutrition Information Per Serving

Calories	360	Protein (g)	16
Fat (g)	14.5	Sodium (mg)	210
Fiber (g)	12.5	Carbohydrates (g)	45
		Cholesterol (mg)	0

Greek Roasted New Potatoes

Serves 6

24 new potatoes (about the size
   of an egg)—allow 3 or 4 per
   person
¼ cup olive oil
2 to 3 T fresh herbs (or 2 to 3 tsp
   dried) such as oregano,
   thyme, and rosemary
Salt and pepper to taste

—Nikki Rose

The simplest and most delicious side dish on earth.

1 Preheat oven to 375°F. Wash and slice the potatoes in half (or quarters if using larger potatoes).

2 Place potatoes in a large, heavy, roasting pan.

3 Sprinkle with olive oil and seasonings, and toss together to blend.

4 Roast for approximately 1 hour, shaking (not stirring) the pan four to five times during baking.

Note: If unable to serve immediately, potatoes can be held in a warm oven (for less than 30 minutes). In the unlikely event of leftovers, toss cold potatoes with a little mustard vinaigrette and serve as a cold salad.

Nutrition Information Per Serving

Calories	345	Protein (g)	7
Fat (g)	9.5	Sodium (mg)	20
Fiber (g)	5.5	Carbohydrates (g)	60
		Cholesterol (mg)	0

Greek Cabbage Salad

—*Nikki Rose*

Serves 6

1 Thinly slice cabbage, and place in a large mixing bowl. Add oil, vinegar, and seasonings, toss together.

2 Marinate for 1 hour before serving.

1 whole cabbage, cleaned and cored

½ cup olive oil

3 T red wine vinegar

Salt and pepper to taste

Nutrition Information Per Serving

Calories 180	Protein (g). 1.6	
Fat (g) 18	Sodium (mg) 25	
Fiber (g). 1.5	Carbohydrates (g) 5	
	Cholesterol (mg). 0	

Lima or Fava Bean Plaki

Serves 8

—Nikki Rose

1 lb dried large white lima beans

½ cup olive oil

1 large onion, diced

4 garlic cloves, minced

2 carrots, diced

2 celery stalks, diced

4 tomatoes, diced

1 lemon, juiced

4 cups nonfat chicken broth or
   vegetable stock

½ cup fresh parsley, chopped

2 T fresh dill, chopped

Salt and pepper to taste

Several different types of beans work well with this recipe. Frozen beans can also be used in a pinch.

1 Soak the lima beans in water overnight; drain, rinse, and add fresh water to cover.

2 Boil for about 30 minutes in a large stockpot; drain and return to the stockpot, and reserve.

3 In a large sauté pan over medium heat, add the olive oil and sauté onions until golden brown. Add garlic, carrots, and celery and sauté 5 minutes more.

4 Combine the above in the stockpot of beans, along with the tomatoes, lemon, and stock.

5 Simmer for about 1 hour or until beans are tender and the stock is reduced to a light sauce.

6 Add the fresh herbs and spices, and simmer for 15 minutes more.

7 Serve hot as a side dish, or cold along with other salads, or at room temperature as a snack with bread. Keeps for 1 week under refrigeration.

Variation: Green Bean Plaki

If you prefer to use green beans instead, make the following adjustments to the recipe:

1 Start with step 3, using a large stockpot.

2 Add 1 lb fresh beans and the remaining ingredients, with only 1 cup of stock instead of 4.

3 Simmer for 30 minutes or less, depending on preference. Serve hot as a side dish, or cold along with other salads, or at room temperature as a snack with bread.

Nutrition Information Per Serving

Calories 360		Protein (g) 16	
Fat (g) 14.5		Sodium (mg) 210	
Fiber (g) 12.5		Carbohydrates (g) 45	
		Cholesterol (mg) 0	

Caponata

—Maxine Clark

Serves 6

A delicious sweet-and-sour eggplant salad, served as an antipasto or as a vegetable. As always in Sicily, serve at room temperature. There are endless variations of this dish; delicious served with beef main dishes.

1 Place the eggplant in a colander; sprinkle with salt, and set aside for 30 minutes.

2 Heat I T olive oil in a saucepan, and add the onion and celery. Cook for 5 minutes until soft but not brown; add the tomatoes and cook for 15 minutes until pulpy. Add all the remaining ingredients and cook for 15 minutes.

3 Rinse and pat the eggplant dry. Deep-fry in olive oil in batches until deep golden brown. Drain well.

4 Stir eggplant into the sauce. Taste and adjust the seasoning. Let stand for at least 30 minutes to allow the flavors to develop before serving. Top with the almonds and parsley. Serve warm.

4 medium eggplants, cut into bite-size cubes

Salt

Olive oil

1 medium onion, chopped

2 celery stalks, sliced

8 ripe red tomatoes, roughly chopped

1 T capers, rinsed well

¼ cup green olives, pitted

3 T red wine vinegar

1 T sugar

Salt and pepper

Toasted, chopped almonds and chopped parsley, for garnish

Nutrition Information Per Serving	
Calories 180	Protein (g) 4.5
Fat (g) 6	Sodium (mg) 195
Fiber (g) 9	Carbohydrates (g) 30
	Cholesterol (mg) 0

Zuppa di Finocchio (Fennel Soup)

Serves 4

—Maxine Clark

¼ cup olive oil

1 medium onion, chopped

1 cup peeled, cored, and thinly
    sliced fennel (Reserve any
    green fronds for garnish.)

1 potato, diced

3 cups nonfat chicken broth

Salt and freshly ground pepper

Fresh lemon juice, to taste

1 Heat olive oil in a large saucepan, and add the onion. Cook for 5 minutes until onion begins to soften.

2 Add fennel and potato, and cook for 5 minutes until fennel begins to soften.

3 Pour in the chicken broth and bring to the boil. Turn down the heat; cover and simmer for about 45 minutes. Puree mixture in a blender, then strain through a sieve.

4 Return mixture to saucepan and reheat. Taste and season well with salt, pepper, and lemon juice. Serve garnished with the reserved fennel fronds.

Nutrition Information Per Serving	
Calories 210	Protein (g) 5.5
Fat (g) 14.5	Sodium (mg) 280
Fiber (g) 1.5	Carbohydrates (g) 17.5
	Cholesterol (mg) 0

Ants on the Trees

—Lan Tan

1 Soak cellophane noodles in warm water for about 5 minutes. Drain and cut into 4-inch sections.

2 Combine ingredients for marinade in a bowl large enough to hold the ground meat. Add the chicken or pork and marinate in refrigerator for about 30 minutes.

3 Combine soy sauce, pepper, and chicken broth for the seasoning sauce, and set aside.

4 Heat oil in wok; add ginger and hot bean sauce. Stir for a few seconds. Add marinated ground chicken or pork. Stir-fry until the meat separates, about 2 minutes. Add the seasoning sauce and cellophane noodles. Mix well. Cover and bring to a boil. Simmer for about 2 minutes, stirring once. Garnish with chopped scallions and sesame oil.

Serves 4

4 oz cellophane noodles
½ lb ground chicken or pork

Marinade:

1 tsp low-sodium soy sauce
2 tsp rice wine
1 tsp cornstarch

Seasoning sauce:

1 tsp low-sodium soy sauce
Pinch white pepper
¾ cup nonfat chicken broth

2 tsp vegetable oil
1 tsp minced ginger
1 tsp low-sodium hot bean sauce
1 T chopped scallions
1 tsp sesame oil

Nutrition Information Per Serving			
Calories	240	Protein (g)	18
Fat (g)	6.5	Sodium (mg)	155
Fiber (g)	1.5	Carbohydrates (g)	25
		Cholesterol (mg)	55

Egg Fu Yung

—Lan Tan

¼ lb boneless, skinless chicken
    breast, or shelled, deveined
    shrimp

Marinade:

1 tsp low-sodium soy sauce

1 tsp rice wine

½ tsp cornstarch

1 ½ tsp peanut or vegetable oil

1 cup diced Chinese cabbage

6 to 8 water chestnuts, diced

1 tsp minced shallots

1 cup fresh bean sprouts

1 tsp low-sodium soy sauce

5 egg whites

Sauce (Optional):

½ cup nonfat chicken broth

1 tsp low-sodium soy sauce

Pinch white pepper

Pinch sugar

1 ½ tsp cornstarch

1 tsp peanut or vegetable oil

Sesame oil

1 T chopped scallions

1 Dice the chicken or shrimp into small pieces.

2 Combine ingredients for marinade. Add the chicken pieces and marinate in refrigerator for about 30 minutes.

3 Heat 1 ½ tsp oil in wok. Stir-fry chicken for 1 minute. Add cabbage, water chestnuts, and shallots. Stir-fry for about 2 minutes. Add bean sprouts. Mix in soy sauce. Stir well. Remove from heat; set aside.

4 Lightly beat egg whites in large bowl. Add all cooked ingredients and mix well. Set aside.

5 If making the sauce, do so now. Heat sauce ingredients in small saucepan, stirring until thickened. Set aside.

6 Heat 1 tsp oil in wok or Dutch oven until hot. Lower heat to medium. Gently ladle in about ½ cup of egg mixture. Fry until golden brown. Fold over with spatula and cook the other side until golden brown. Remove each cooked portion to hot platter in warm oven. Repeat with remaining ingredients.

7 Serve with or without sauce. Garnish with drops of sesame oil and chopped scallions.

Nutrition Information Per Serving	
Calories 270	Protein (g) 20
Fat (g) 10	Sodium (mg) 330
Fiber (g) . . . . >1	Carbohydrates (g) 30
	Cholesterol (mg) 20

Chicken Fried Rice

—Lan Tan

1 Prepare marinade; set aside.

2 Cut the chicken cutlet into thin strips. Add to the marinade and let sit for about 30 minutes in refrigerator.

3 Heat 1 tsp oil in wok or Dutch oven. Stir-fry chicken for about 2 minutes or until chicken turns white. Remove and set aside.

4 Heat 1 tsp. oil in wok or Dutch oven. Stir in beaten egg. Scramble and break into small pieces. Remove and set aside.

5 Heat 2 tsp oil in wok or Dutch oven. Stir-fry half the scallions until lightly browned, about 1 minute.

6 Add rice and stir until the rice is separate and thoroughly heated. Add soy sauce and white pepper. Mix well. Add scrambled egg, bean sprouts, and cooked chicken. Stir until well blended. Garnish with remaining chopped scallions.

Marinade:

1 tsp low-sodium soy sauce

2 tsp rice wine

½ tsp cornstarch

Pinch white pepper

¼ lb boneless, skinless chicken breast

1 T peanut or vegetable oil

1 egg, lightly beaten

2 T finely chopped scallions

3½ cups cooked rice

1½ T low-sodium soy sauce

¼ tsp white pepper

1 cup bean sprouts, rinsed and drained

Nutrition Information Per Serving	
Calories 200	Protein (g) 9
Fat (g) 3.5	Sodium (mg) 175
Fiber (g) . . . . <1	Carbohydrates (g) 30
	Cholesterol (mg) 40

Healthy Kung Pao Chicken

Serves 4

—Lan Tan

Marinade:

1 tsp low-sodium soy sauce

2 tsp rice wine

1 tsp cornstarch

$\frac{1}{2}$ lb boneless, skinless chicken breast, cut into $\frac{1}{2}$-inch cubes

Sauce:

2 T low-sodium soy sauce

1 T rice wine

2 tsp sugar

1 tsp black vinegar

1 tsp cornstarch mixed with 1 T nonfat chicken broth

1 tsp sesame oil

2 T peanut or vegetable oil

8 dried red peppers, or to taste

1 T finely chopped ginger

1 tsp chili paste with garlic

$\frac{1}{2}$ cup chopped green bell pepper

$\frac{1}{2}$ cup chopped red bell pepper

$\frac{1}{2}$ cup chopped bamboo shoots

$\frac{1}{4}$ cup diced water chestnuts

2 T finely chopped scallions

$\frac{1}{4}$ cup raw peanuts (optional)

1 In small bowl, combine marinade ingredients. Add cubed chicken and toss to coat. Cover with plastic wrap and refrigerate for 30 minutes.

2 Combine sauce ingredients in a small bowl; set aside.

3 Heat 1 T oil in wok or Dutch oven. Stir the diced chicken until it turns white, about 2 minutes. Remove and set aside. Wipe out wok.

4 Heat 1 T oil in wok. Add the dried peppers, chopped ginger, and chili paste with garlic. Stir for a few seconds. Add red and green bell peppers, bamboo shoots, and water chestnuts. Stir and mix well; cook 1 minute. Add the sauce. Mix thoroughly and cook 1 minute, stirring until it thickens. Add the cooked chicken and scallions, and cook 1 minute longer. Stir in the raw peanuts (optional). Serve immediately.

Nutrition Information Per Serving with $\frac{1}{2}$ Cup Cooked White Rice

Calories	295	Protein (g)	17
Fat (g)	9	Sodium (mg)	345
Fiber (g)	1	Carbohydrates (g)	35
		Cholesterol (mg)	35

Moo Shu Chicken with Pancakes

—Lan Tan

1 Prepare marinade. Add chicken and let set in refrigerator for 30 minutes.

2 Heat I T oil in wok or Dutch oven. Add half of the scallions, then the chicken, and stir-fry over high heat until chicken turns white, about 2 minutes. Add I T hoisin sauce. Mix well. Remove and set aside.

3 Heat 2 tsp oil in wok. Add cabbage, tree ears, mushrooms, lily flowers, and bamboo shoots. Stir-fry until the cabbage softens, about 4 minutes. Add 2 tsp soy sauce, the cooked chicken, and the remaining scallions. Garnish with sesame oil. Cook until chicken is heated through, about I minute.

4 Spread a thin layer of hoisin sauce on *moo shu* pancakes or flour tortillas, and fill with chicken-vegetable mixture. Roll up the pancake.

Marinade:

2 tsp low-sodium soy sauce

2 tsp rice wine

1 ½ tsp cornstarch

½ lb boneless, skinless chicken breast, julienned

2 T peanut or vegetable oil

2 T finely sliced scallions

1 T hoisin sauce

1 cup thinly sliced Chinese cabbage, stems only

2 T (1 large) tree ears, soaked in warm water for 20 minutes and drained, with tough stems removed and thinly sliced

4 to 6 dried mushrooms, soaked in warm water for 20 minutes, drained and coarsely chopped

¼ cup dried lily flowers, soaked in warm water for 20 minutes, drained and coarsely chopped

½ cup coarsely chopped bamboo shoots

2 tsp low-sodium soy sauce

1 tsp sesame oil

4 to 8 *moo shu* pancakes,* or substitute flour tortillas

Hoisin sauce for garnish

Available at Asian markets.

Nutrition Information Per Serving with One *Moo Shu* Pancake

Calories	320	Protein (g)	18.5
Fat (g)	12	Sodium (mg)	310
Fiber (g)	3.5	Carbohydrates (g)	35
		Cholesterol (mg)	35

Chicken with Cashews in Hoisin Sauce

Serves 4

Marinade:

2 tsp low-sodium soy sauce

2 tsp rice wine

1 tsp cornstarch

½ lb boneless, skinless chicken
    breast

4 to 6 dried black mushrooms

8 to 10 water chestnuts

½ cup bamboo shoots

Vegetable oil

1 tsp finely chopped ginger

1 tsp finely chopped garlic

1 T hoisin sauce

½ T chopped scallions

1 T cashews, dry-roasted,
    coarsely chopped

—Lan Tan

1 Prepare marinade. Cut chicken into ½-inch cubes, add to marinade, and let sit for 30 minutes in refrigerator.

2 Soak mushrooms in hot water for about 20 minutes. Remove and discard the stems. Dice mushrooms, water chestnuts, and bamboo shoots; set aside.

3 Heat ½ T oil in wok or Dutch oven until very hot. Add ginger and garlic and stir-fry until fragrant, about 10 seconds. Add mushrooms, bamboo shoots, and water chestnuts. Stir and mix well, about 1 minute. Remove and set aside.

4 Heat 1 T oil in wok or Dutch oven; add marinated chicken cubes and stir gently until the chicken turns white, about 2 minutes. Add the cooked mushrooms, water chestnuts, bamboo shoots, and hoisin sauce. Stir thoroughly. Turn off heat. Garnish with scallions and cashews.

Nutrition Information Per Serving with ½ Cup Cooked White Rice

Calories	260	Protein (g)	17
Fat (g)	3.5	Sodium (mg)	45
Fiber (g)	2	Carbohydrates (g)	40
		Cholesterol (mg)	35

Chicken with Broccoli

—Lan Tan

1 Prepare marinade; set aside.

2 Prepare sauce; set aside.

3 Add chicken to marinade and let sit in refrigerator for 30 minutes.

4 Steam broccoli for 2 to 3 minutes. Drain and rinse under cold water; set aside.

5 Heat 2 tsp oil in wok or Dutch oven. Stir-fry ginger and garlic for 1 minute, then add broccoli and stir-fry 1 minute more. Remove from pan; set aside.

6 Heat 1 T oil in wok or Dutch oven. Add chicken and stir until the chicken is almost cooked, about 1½ minutes. Add the seasoning sauce. Mix well. Add broccoli and stir thoroughly; cook 1 minute more until broccoli is heated through and chicken is completely cooked.

Marinade:
2 tsp low-sodium soy sauce
2 tsp rice wine
½ tsp cornstarch

Sauce:
2 tsp low-sodium soy sauce
1 T oyster sauce
2 tsp rice wine
1 tsp sesame oil
Pinch white pepper
1 tsp cornstarch mixed with
    ¼ cup nonfat chicken broth

½ lb boneless, skinless chicken
    breast, julienned
¾ lb broccoli, cut into florets,
    stems peeled and sliced
    diagonally into ¼-inch slices
Vegetable oil
½ tsp grated ginger
1 garlic clove, coarsely chopped

Nutrition Information Per Serving with ½ Cup Cooked White Rice			
Calories	265	Protein (g)	19
Fat (g)	6	Sodium (mg)	345
Fiber (g)	3	Carbohydrates (g)	35
		Cholesterol (mg)	35

Chicken in Garlic Sauce

Serves 4

—Lan Tan

Marinade:

2 tsp low-sodium soy sauce

1 tsp rice wine

1 tsp cornstarch

Sauce:

2 T low-sodium soy sauce

1 tsp rice wine

2 tsp sugar

1 ½ tsp black vinegar

1 tsp sesame oil

⅛ tsp white pepper

1 tsp cornstarch

2 T nonfat chicken broth

½ lb boneless, skinless chicken
    breast, cut into thin strips

2 T dried tree ears

1 ½ T peanut or vegetable oil

½ tsp coarsely chopped ginger

garlic clove, coarsely chopped

1 tsp chili paste with garlic

12 water chestnuts, diced

1 T coarsely chopped scallions

1 Prepare marinade; set aside.

2 Prepare sauce; set aside.

3 Marinate chicken in marinade for 30 minutes in refrigerator.

4 Soak the tree ears in hot water for 20 minutes. Wash carefully, then dice them into small pieces.

5 Heat I T oil over high heat in wok or Dutch oven. Stir-fry the marinated chicken for about 2 minutes or until chicken turns white. Remove from pan and set aside.

6 Heat ½ T of oil in wok or Dutch oven. Add ginger, garlic, and chili paste. Stir-fry for a few seconds. Add tree ears and water chestnuts. Stir and mix well. Add the seasoning sauce. Stir until thick, about I minute. Add cooked chicken and mix thoroughly. Cook about I minute more until chicken is heated through. Turn off heat. Garnish with chopped scallions.

Nutrition Information Per Serving with ½ Cup Cooked White Rice

Calories	315	Protein (g)	17.5
Fat (g)	7	Sodium (mg)	360
Fiber (g)	2	Carbohydrates (g)	45
		Cholesterol (mg)	35

Moo Goo Gai Pan

—Lan Tan

1 Prepare marinade; set aside.

2 Combine the sauce ingredients in a small bowl; set aside.

3 Marinate chicken in soy sauce marinade for 30 minutes in refrigerator.

4 Soak the tree ears in hot water for 15 minutes, then wash carefully.

5 Cut the snow peas diagonally and the baby corn in half lengthwise.

6 Heat 1 T oil in wok or Dutch oven over high heat until hot. Stir-fry the garlic and ginger until fragrant, about 10 seconds. Add chicken and continuously stir until the chicken turns white, about 2 minutes. Set aside.

7 Heat 1 T oil in the wok or Dutch oven. Add scallions, tree ears, straw mushrooms, and baby corn, and stir for a few seconds. Stir in the seasoning sauce, then the cornstarch mix. Bring liquid to a boil; stir constantly, about 1 minute or until it thickens. Add the snow peas and cooked chicken. Mix thoroughly and cook about 1 minute until chicken and snow peas are heated through.

Marinade:

1 T low-sodium soy sauce

½ T rice wine

1 tsp cornstarch

Sauce:

2 tsp oyster sauce

2 tsp rice wine

1 tsp sesame oil

⅛ tsp sugar

⅛ tsp white pepper

1 cup nonfat chicken broth

½ lb boneless, skinless chicken
   breast, julienned

1 T dried tree ears (or 1 small)

¼ lb snow peas, steamed until
   tender crisp, about 2
   minutes, and then rinsed
   under cold running water

Vegetable oil

1 garlic clove, finely chopped

1 tsp finely chopped ginger

2 scallions, chopped

¾ cup straw mushrooms, or 6
   dried mushrooms, soaked in
   hot water until softened,
   then rinsed and thinly sliced

½ cup baby corn (optional)

1 T cornstarch mixed with 2 T
   nonfat chicken broth

Nutrition Information Per Serving with ½ Cup Cooked White Rice	
Calories 285	Protein (g) 20
Fat (g) 6	Sodium (mg) 355
Fiber (g) 2	Carbohydrates (g) 35
	Cholesterol (mg) 35

Orange-Flavored Chicken

Serves 4

—Lan Tan

Marinade:

2 tsp low-sodium soy sauce

2 tsp rice wine

1 tsp cornstarch

Sauce:

2 T orange juice

1 T low-sodium soy sauce

2 tsp rice wine

2 tsp ketchup

2 tsp sugar

1 tsp sesame oil

Pinch white pepper

1 tsp cornstarch mixed with 3 T
   nonfat chicken broth

½ lb boneless, skinless chicken
   breast, julienned

Vegetable oil

2 tsp chopped ginger

6 dried red peppers

1 tsp grated orange rind (1–2
   oranges)

1 T chopped scallions

1 Prepare marinade; set aside.

2 Combine the sauce ingredients; set aside.

3 Marinate chicken in soy sauce marinade for about 1 hour in refrigerator.

4 Heat 1 T oil in wok or Dutch oven until hot. Add chicken. Stir-fry for about 2 minutes until chicken turns white. Remove and set aside.

5 Heat 2 tsp oil in wok until hot. Add chopped ginger, dried red peppers, and grated orange peel. Stir-fry for about 1 minute, then add seasoning sauce. Stir until thick. Add cooked chicken. Mix thoroughly; cook about 1 minute until chicken is heated through. Turn off heat. Garnish with scallions.

Nutrition Information Per Serving with ½ Cup Cooked White Rice	
Calories 220	Protein (g) 16
Fat (g) 2.5	Sodium (mg) 235
Fiber (g) . . . . >1	Carbohydrates (g) 30
	Cholesterol (mg) 35

Stir-fried Tofu with Chicken and Vegetables

—Kyoko Konishi

1 Drain tofu and coarsely crumble.

2 Slice carrot into thin strips.

3 Soak dried mushrooms in hot water until softened, about 20 minutes. Drain, remove and discard tough stems, and cut caps into thin strips.

4 Mix together soy sauce, rice wine, and sugar; set aside.

5 In a wok or large nonstick skillet, heat the oil over medium-high heat until hot but not smoking.

6 Add the ginger and cook until fragrant, about 10 seconds.

7 Add the ground chicken and stir-fry until the meat turns white, about 2 minutes.

8 Add the carrots and mushrooms and continue to cook until the carrots are tender, about 2 minutes longer.

9 Add the tofu and gently mix.

10 Stir in the soy sauce mixture and scallion slices, and cook until the tofu is heated through, about 1 minute.

11 Mix in the egg and cook for about 1 minute longer. Remove from heat and serve.

One 14-oz container firm, light tofu

1 large carrot

4 dried shiitake mushrooms

3 T low-sodium soy sauce

2 T rice wine

1 T sugar

1 ½ T vegetable oil

1 tsp finely minced ginger

¼ lb ground chicken

2 scallions, cut into ½-inch slices

1 large egg, lightly beaten

Nutrition Information Per Serving

Calories 310		Protein (g) 20	
Fat (g) 9.8		Sodium (mg) 595	
Fiber (g) 1.5		Carbohydrates (g) 35	
		Cholesterol (mg) 70	

Soba Noodles with Chicken and Mushrooms

Serves 4

—Francine Fielding

2 tsp rice wine

2 tsp low-sodium soy sauce

½ lb boneless, skinless chicken breasts, cut into thin strips

3 to 4 dried shiitake mushrooms

8 oz soba noodles

4 cups dashi

3 T mirin

2 T low-sodium soy sauce

One 4-oz package enoki mushrooms, bottom 2 to 3 inches trimmed off

¼ cup finely chopped scallions

1 In a small glass or ceramic bowl, combine the rice wine and soy sauce. Add the chicken and toss well to coat with the marinade. Cover with plastic wrap and refrigerate for 10 minutes.

2 Soak the dried mushrooms in hot water until softened, about 20 minutes. Drain. Remove and discard tough stems, and slice caps into thin strips.

3 Cook the soba noodles in boiling water until just tender, about 5 minutes. Drain. Rinse with warm water.

4 In a large pot, combine dashi, mirin, and soy sauce. Bring to a gentle boil over medium-high heat.

5 Add the chicken. Reduce the heat to a simmer and cook until the meat turns white, about 3 to 4 minutes. Skim off foam that may float to the top.

6 Add the shiitake mushrooms and the enoki mushrooms and simmer for 1 minute.

7 Add the soba noodles and cook for 1 minute longer.

8 Divide the soup and noodles among four bowls, and sprinkle each with 1 T of the chopped scallions.

Nutrition Information Per Serving

Calories	460	Protein (g)	30
Fat (g)	5	Sodium (mg)	2440
Fiber (g)	3	Carbohydrates (g)	75
		Cholesterol (mg)	35

Oyaka Donburi

—Francine Fielding

Serves 4

1 In a small glass or ceramic bowl, whisk together rice wine and soy sauce. Add chicken slices and toss to coat with the marinade. Cover with plastic wrap and refrigerate for 20 minutes.

2 In a large flat-bottomed skillet or sauté pan, combine the dashi, soy sauce, mirin, and sugar. Bring to a boil over medium-high heat.

3 Add the onion slices; reduce heat to a simmer and cook the onion for 1 minute. Add the chicken and simmer until it turns white, about 2 to 3 minutes.

4 Pour the eggs gently into the simmering liquid and cook for 2 minutes without stirring. Stir the eggs. At this point, the eggs will still be a little runny and can be cooked longer, if desired.

5 Divide hot rice among four bowls. Gently spoon the egg mixture over the rice. Garnish each with chopped scallions.

1 tsp rice wine

1 tsp low-sodium soy sauce

¼ lb skinless, boneless chicken breast, cut into thin strips

1 cup dashi

3 T low-sodium soy sauce

2 T mirin

1 T sugar

1 small onion, cut in half, then cut into thin slices (1 cup)

4 eggs, lightly beaten or 1 cup egg substitute

4 cups hot cooked white rice

2 T finely chopped scallions

Nutrition Information Per Serving	
Calories 415	Protein (g) 20
Fat (g) 6	Sodium (mg) 990
Fiber (g) 2	Carbohydrates (g) 65
	Cholesterol (mg) 200

Sautéed Chicken Breasts with Roasted Garlic Sauce

Serves 4

4 boneless skinless chicken
   breasts
¼ cup olive oil
1 garlic clove, minced
2 T fresh rosemary or 1 T dried
   rosemary
1 large head of garlic
½ cup dry white wine
1 sprig of fresh rosemary
¼ cup nonfat chicken stock
Salt and pepper

—— Francis Trzeciak

1 Marinate chicken breasts in olive oil, minced garlic, and rosemary overnight or at least 2 hours.

2 Preheat oven to 350°F. Slice off the top of the garlic head and lightly sprinkle it with olive oil. Roast garlic for about 1 hour, or until soft and golden brown. Set garlic aside to cool, but leave oven on for chicken breasts.

3 When garlic has cooled, squeeze out garlic pulp, mash, and set aside.

4 Sauté chicken in olive oil, a couple of minutes each side. Put in oven for about 15 minutes.

5 Boil wine, 1 sprig of fresh rosemary, mashed roasted garlic, and chicken stock. Add salt and pepper to taste. Leave on high heat until sauce thickens. Strain through fine sieve or put in blender/food processor at high speed (remove rosemary first).

6 Place one chicken breast on each plate and pour sauce over chicken. Garnish with rosemary sprig.

Nutrition Information Per Serving

Calories	320	Protein (g)	55
Fat (g)	6.5	Sodium (mg)	150
Fiber (g)	>1	Carbohydrates (g)	3.5
		Cholesterol (mg)	145

Swedish Cheese-Stuffed Chicken Breasts

—Birgitta Rasmusson

Serves 4

1 Make a slit in chicken breasts, and fill with cheese and celery; secure with toothpicks.

2 In medium pan, sauté chicken in oil over medium-high heat until nearly cooked through (chicken should be barely pink on the inside). Season with salt and pepper.

3 Pour chicken stock and wine over the chicken breasts and let boil for 8 to 10 minutes until chicken is thoroughly cooked.

4 Mix cornstarch with 1 T water and pour in the pan. Let cook for 1 minute. Serve with pasta or rice and vegetables.

4 skinless, boneless chicken breasts

1.5 oz strongly flavored cheese such as bleu

2 celery stalks, finely chopped

1 T vegetable oil

Salt and pepper

3/4 cup nonfat chicken broth

1/3 cup white wine

1 T cornstarch

Nutrition Information Per Serving

Calories 380	Protein (g) 55
Fat (g) 13	Sodium (mg) 360
Fiber (g) . . . . >1	Carbohydrates (g) 3
	Cholesterol (mg) 155

Sicilian Lemon Chicken

Serves 6

3 ½ lb free-range chicken

4 lemons

8 garlic cloves

1 to 2 small red chilies

1 T honey

4 T chopped fresh parsley

Salt and pepper

—Maxine Clark

Chicken pieces are marinated in lemon juice, chilis, and garlic, with a touch of honey to help brown the chicken skin during cooking. Ripe, juicy lemon halves are tucked in and around the joints to impart extra flavor during roasting.

1 Using a sharp knife and/or poultry shears, cut the whole chicken into 8 small or 4 large pieces. Place chicken parts skin-side down in a large, shallow, ovenproof baking dish.

2 Halve the lemons; squeeze the juice and pour into a small bowl; reserve the lemon halves.

3 Peel and crush two of the garlic cloves and add to the lemon juice. Halve the chili(es) lengthwise and remove the seeds. Add to the lemon juice with the honey. Stir well and pour over the chicken. Tuck the lemon halves around chicken pieces. Cover and leave to marinate for at least 2 hours, turning once or twice.

4 Preheat the oven to 400°F. Turn the chicken skin-side up. Halve the rest of the garlic cloves and scatter over the chicken. Roast for 45 minutes or until golden brown and tender. Season with salt and pepper to taste. Serve hot, garnished with the parsley and roasted lemon halves.

Nutrition Information Per Serving

Calories	260	Protein (g)	35
Fat (g)	8.5	Sodium (mg)	95
Fiber (g)	>1	Carbohydrates (g)	9.5
		Cholesterol (mg)	110

Domodah (Groundnut Chicken Stew)

—Hope Farrell

Serves 4 to 6

This dish is traditionally made with chicken pieces with the skin. To save fat and calories, skinless chicken breasts are used. A complete meal.

1 Wash and dry chicken and trim visible fat. Heat peanut oil in a large heavy pot or Dutch oven. Brown the chicken on all sides, a few pieces at a time.

2 While the chicken is browning, place onions, tomatoes, garlic, and chili pepper in a food processor and pulse until finely chopped, or mince all by hand.

3 Heat 1 cup chicken broth and stir slowly into the peanut butter and tomato paste until smooth.

4 When all the chicken has been browned, pour off the oil in the pot and discard. Add onion-tomato mixture, peanut butter mixture, pepper flakes if using, remaining 2 cups chicken broth, tomato juice, salt, and white pepper to the pot and stir to blend. Return the chicken to the pot, bring to a simmer, and cook for 30 minutes.

5 While the chicken is simmering, cut carrots on the diagonal into ¼-inch slices. Wash and slice the eggplant in half lengthwise. Remove stem and cut eggplant halves into ¼-inch slices. Wash okra and trim off caps.

6 When the chicken has simmered for 30 minutes, taste sauce and add salt or pepper if necessary. Add carrots, eggplant, and okra to the pot and simmer all for another 15 minutes, or until vegetables are tender. Serve over rice.

3 pounds of chicken breast
    halves, skinless

2 T peanut oil

2 large onions (¾ lb), quartered

4 large tomatoes, skinned,
    seeded, and cored

2 garlic cloves

1 3-inch hot chili pepper, seeded,
    or ½ tsp red pepper flakes

3 cups nonfat chicken broth,
    divided

1 cup smooth, natural peanut
    butter (without sweeteners)

2 T tomato paste

2 cups tomato juice

1 tsp salt

½ tsp white pepper

3 large carrots, peeled

1 small eggplant (¾ lb)

½ lb fresh okra

4 to 6 cups cooked rice

Nutrition Information Per Serving

Calories 1280	Protein (g) 70
Fat (g) 30	Sodium (mg) 1225
Fiber (g) 11.5	Carbohydrates (g) 180
	Cholesterol (mg) 105

Chicken Yassa

Serves 4

—Hope Farrell

Four 5 to 6 oz boneless, skinless
  chicken breasts (1 ¼ to 1 ½
  lbs total)

¼ cup peanut oil, divided

½ cup freshly squeezed lemon
  juice

4 large garlic cloves, minced
  (1 T)

1 tsp fresh, grated ginger

1 3-inch hot chili pepper, seeded
  and minced, or ½ tsp red
  pepper flakes

1 ½ tsp ground black pepper

1 tsp salt

4 large onions, thinly sliced
  (1 ¼ lbs) (5 cups)

Parsley, lemon slices, or chili
  pepper rings for garnish
  (optional)

3 to 4 cups cooked white rice

1 Preheat the grill or broiler.

2 Trim chicken breasts of any fat or gristle. Place in a glass bowl. Mix 3 tablespoons peanut oil, the lemon juice, garlic, ginger, chili pepper, black pepper, and salt. Pour the oil mixture over the chicken and marinate for 30 minutes, turning chicken after 15 minutes.

3 While the chicken is marinating, heat the remaining teaspoon of oil in a nonstick frying pan. Sauté the onions over medium heat for 25 minutes, stirring often, until tender and golden.

4 Remove the chicken breasts from the marinade and reserve marinade. Grill chicken 5 to 6 minutes per side, or until cooked through. Meanwhile, add reserved marinade to the onions and simmer for 5 minutes. Taste onions and add additional black or red pepper if more heat is desired. Set onions aside and keep warm.

5 When chicken is done, place on a hot platter or plates; cover with the sautéed onions; garnish, and serve with rice.

Nutrition Information Per Serving			
Calories	620	Protein (g)	45
Fat (g)	16	Sodium (mg)	650
Fiber (g)	3.5	Carbohydrates (g)	70
		Cholesterol (mg)	100

Vegetable Lo Mein

—Lan Tan

Serves 4

1 Combine sauce ingredients in a small bowl; set aside.

2 Drop noodles in boiling water for about 3 minutes. Drain and rinse under cold running water. Mix with 2 tsp vegetable oil. Set aside.

3 Soak the mushrooms in hot water for about 20 minutes. Remove and discard tough stems. Shred mushroom caps into long, thin strips.

4 Heat 1½ T oil in wok or Dutch oven until hot. Stir-fry scallions for about 1 minute. Add snow peas and carrots and stir for 1 minute more. Add cabbage, black mushrooms, and ½ cup bean sprouts. Stir and mix well.

5 Spread the cooked noodles on the vegetable mixture. Add the seasoning sauce. Toss over high heat for a few minutes until noodles are heated through. Add remaining 1 cup bean sprouts. Mix thoroughly.

Sauce:

1 T low-sodium soy sauce

1 tsp oyster sauce

1 tsp sesame oil

⅛ tsp white pepper

8 oz fresh or dried lo mein noodles

2 tsp vegetable oil

4 dried black mushrooms

1½ T peanut or vegetable oil

1 stalk scallion, split in half lengthwise, cut into 1-inch pieces

½ cup (2 oz) thinly sliced snow peas

¼ cup thinly sliced carrots

1 cup shredded Chinese cabbage

1½ cups bean sprouts

Nutrition Information Per Serving			
Calories	335	Protein (g)	11
Fat (g)	10	Sodium (mg)	270
Fiber (g)	4	Carbohydrates (g)	50
		Cholesterol (mg)	55

Crispy Asian Tofu

Serves 4

—*Anne Patterson*

1 lb frozen water-packed extra-firm tofu, thawed*

¾ cup water

2 T low-sodium soy sauce

1 T rice vinegar

3 garlic cloves, finely minced

1 T brown sugar

1 ½ cups soft, finely ground, whole-wheat bread crumbs

½ tsp salt

½ tsp Chinese Five-Spice Powder†

4 T flour

1 tsp dark sesame oil plus 2 tsp vegetable oil

*To freeze water-packed tofu, drain water from package, wrap in heavy-duty aluminum foil and freeze for at least 2 days. Tofu may be frozen up to 4 months. Thaw in refrigerator just like any perishable item. Or, it can be unwrapped and defrosted in the microwave.

†Found with other spices in the supermarket. Chinese Five-Spice Powder is a blend of cinnamon, star anise, anise seed, ginger, and cloves. Wonderful for stir-frying.

1 Wrap thawed tofu in a tea towel and gently squeeze out water. The tofu will be caramel colored, and the texture will be thick and spongy. Cut tofu lengthwise into 4 long slices, then cut each slice into three equal pieces for 12 pieces total.

2 In a shallow glass dish, stir together water, soy sauce, rice vinegar, garlic, and brown sugar for the marinade.

3 Add tofu and turn to cover. Marinate for 10 minutes.

4 In a shallow bowl, combine the bread crumbs, salt, and Five-Spice Powder. Place the flour in another small bowl.

5 Remove tofu slices from marinade and dip each piece in flour; dip back into marinade, then dip in bread crumb mixture, covering all sides.

6 In a large nonstick skillet, heat sesame and vegetable oils on medium-high heat until hot, but not smoking.

7 Cook tofu until golden brown, about 2 minutes. Gently turn and cook on all remaining sides until golden, about 1 minute per side. Serve over stir-fried vegetables.

Nutrition Information Per Serving

Calories	250	Protein (g)	15
Fat (g)	6.9	Sodium (mg)	1010
Fiber (g)	4.5	Carbohydrates (g)	35
		Cholesterol (mg)	0

Mediterranean Rice Pilaf

—Lynn Kutner

—Lynn Kutner

Serves 6 to 8

1 Toast pignoli nuts in a dry pan over medium heat, stirring constantly until they brown. *Beware:* They burn easily. Remove immediately to a bowl.

2 In a heavy pot, sauté onion in butter to soften. Add rice and stir 2 minutes.

3 Add boiling liquid, salt, pepper, and saffron. Stir once; cover. Simmer 18 to 20 minutes. Remove from heat. Let stand 2 to 3 minutes covered before fluffing with pignolis and chopped herbs.

½ cup pignoli (pine) nuts

2 medium onions (or 1 large)

2 T butter (or butter and olive oil mixed)

2 cups Carolina rice

4 cups boiling liquid (choice of water, chicken stock, or half chicken stock, half water)

½ to 1 ½ tsp salt (depending on saltiness; start with lesser amount, unless you use all water)

Pinch pepper

½ tsp saffron threads

2 to 3 T fresh chopped parsley or mint

Nutrition Information Per Serving			
Calories	250	Protein (g)	5.5
Fat (g)	7	Sodium (mg)	33
Fiber (g)	2	Carbohydrates (g)	40
		Cholesterol (mg)	8

Eggplant Szechuan Style

Serves 4

—Lan Tan

Sauce:

¼ cup nonfat chicken or vegetable broth

1½ T low-sodium soy sauce

1 T rice wine

2 tsp sugar

1 tsp rice vinegar

1 lb eggplant

1 T vegetable oil

1 garlic clove, finely chopped

1 tsp grated fresh ginger

1 tsp low-sodium chili paste with garlic

2 tsp sweet bean sauce

1 tsp cornstarch mixed with 1 T water

1 tsp sesame oil

1 stalk scallions, chopped

Black pepper, to taste

1 Prepare seasoning sauce; set aside.

2 Wash and drain eggplant. Cut in half lengthwise. Cut each half into ¼-inch slices crosswise (half-moons).

3 Steam the eggplant over boiling water for about 8 to 10 minutes or until soft. Remove and set aside.

4 In a large nonstick skillet or wok, heat oil over high heat until hot but not smoking. Add garlic, ginger, chili paste, and sweet bean sauce and cook for about 10 seconds or until fragrant.

5 Add cooked eggplant and sauce. Mix well and bring to a boil. Add cornstarch and stir until mixture thickens, about 1 minute. Garnish with sesame oil and chopped scallions, and season with pepper.

Nutrition Information Per Serving

Calories 95	Protein (g) 2
Fat (g) 5	Sodium (mg) 255
Fiber (g) 3	Carbohydrates (g) 10
	Cholesterol (mg) 0

Tofu-Basil Pasta Sauce on Fettuccine

—Anne Patterson

Serves 4

1 In bowl of food processor or blender, blend tofu until smooth. Blend in onion, white pepper, and I T basil.

2 In large skillet, heat oil over medium heat. Add minced garlic and sauté I minute.

3 Turn heat to low and add the blended tofu mixture. Stir in Parmesan cheese and cook 2 to 3 minutes, stirring constantly over low heat until cheese melts. Add milk and stir. Season with salt and pepper. Serve immediately over cooked pasta. Garnish with remaining I T chopped basil.

10.5 oz light, silken-soft tofu, drained

1 tsp finely chopped onion

1/4 tsp white pepper

2 T chopped fresh basil

1 T vegetable oil

2 garlic cloves, minced

1/2 cup freshly grated Parmesan

2 T plain, light soy milk or regular milk

Salt and pepper, to taste

4 cups cooked fettuccine

Nutrition Information Per Serving			
Calories	310	Protein (g)	16.5
Fat (g)	8	Sodium (mg)	265
Fiber (g)	2	Carbohydrates (g)	40
		Cholesterol (mg)	10

Eggplant and Green Pepper Stir-Fry with Miso Sauce

Serves 4

—*Francine Fielding*

½ lb Japanese eggplant

1 large green bell pepper

½ cup water

2 T low-sodium soy sauce

2 T rice wine

2 T mirin

2 T white miso

2 tsp sugar

1 tsp cornstarch dissolved in 1 T water

1 T vegetable oil

1 tsp finely minced ginger

2 cups cooked rice

1 Slice eggplant in half lengthwise, then into ⅛-inch-thick slices crosswise. Soak in cold water for 5 minutes, then drain.

2 Slice green pepper into ½-inch squares.

3 Combine the water, soy sauce, rice wine, mirin, miso, and sugar in a small bowl. Mix well to make sure the sugar is dissolved. Set aside.

4 Mix the cornstarch with water and set aside.

5 In a wok or large nonstick skillet, heat the oil over medium-high heat until hot but not smoking. Add the ginger, and stir-fry until fragrant, about 10 seconds.

6 Add the eggplant and stir-fry for 3 minutes.

7 Add the green peppers and cook for 2 minutes longer or until the vegetables are tender. Add the sauce mixture and mix well.

8 Stir in cornstarch and simmer, stirring constantly until sauce thickens, about 1 minute. Serve with rice.

Nutrition Information Per Serving with ½ Cup Cooked White Rice

Calories 220		Protein (g) 4.5	
Fat (g) 4.5		Sodium (mg) 615	
Fiber (g) 2		Carbohydrates (g) 35	
		Cholesterol (mg) 0	

Vegetable Sushi Rolls

——Francine Fielding

Serves 6

1 Rinse the rice under cold running water until water runs clear. Place rice, water, and rice wine in a pot, uncovered, and bring to a gentle boil. Cover and lower heat to low. Cook for 15 to 20 minutes until all liquid is evaporated. Turn off heat and let sit for 5 minutes.

2 Mix rice vinegar, sugar, and salt.

3 Place rice in a large shallow bowl or on a large platter. Pour the rice vinegar mixture over the rice. Using a spatula, turn the rice over to mix in the seasoning and to quickly cool down the rice. Continue to mix the rice until the liquid is absorbed.

4 Fold in the chopped scallions. Spread the rice mixture thinly in the bowl to help it cool down. Set aside until rice cools.

5 Place 1 nori sheet, shiny-side down, on a bamboo sushi-rolling mat.

6 With moistened hands, spread ¼ of the rice thinly over the sheet, leaving a ½-inch strip at the top end.

7 Spread a little of the wasabi paste on a strip along the center of the rice.

8 Spread some of each vegetable along the center, making sure there is some of each vegetable across the whole sheet. Starting at the end nearest you, roll the nori sheet over the vegetables to enclose them; then continue to roll the nori tightly. Moisten the ½-inch strip with a little water to seal the roll.

9 Place seam side down on a platter and continue with the remaining nori sheets. Cut each strip into 6 to 8 slices and arrange on a platter.

10 Serve with wasabi paste, soy sauce, and pickled ginger.

Ingredients:

2 cups Japanese rice

2 cups water

1½ T rice wine

¼ cup unseasoned rice vinegar

1 T sugar

½ tsp salt

¼ cup finely chopped scallions

4 nori (toasted seaweed) sheets

wasabi powder mixed with water to make a paste

¼ cup snow peas, blanched and cut into long thin strips

1 large carrot, cut into long, thin strips

1 small red bell pepper, cut into long, thin strips

1 small green bell pepper, cut into long, thin strips

¼ English cucumber, seeded and cut into long, thin strips

Soy sauce

Pickled ginger

Nutrition Information Per Serving			
Calories	300	Protein (g)	6
Fat (g)	>1	Sodium (mg)	355
Fiber (g)	4	Carbohydrates (g)	65
		Cholesterol (mg)	0

Stuffed Tofu Pasta Shells
with Marinara Sauce for a Crowd

Serves 15

—Anne Patterson

Sauce:

1 T vegetable oil

1 medium onion, finely chopped

14 garlic cloves, minced

Four 14.5-oz cans diced
tomatoes

½ tsp ground cumin

½ tsp dried oregano

¼ cup chopped fresh
mushrooms

Filling:

One 10-oz package frozen,
chopped spinach

2 cups (1 ½ lb) firm tofu, drained,
patted dry, and mashed

8 oz part-skim mozzarella
cheese, shredded

1 tsp salt

Pepper to taste

3 egg whites

½ cup grated Parmesan cheese

1 lb dry jumbo macaroni shells,
cooked and drained

1 Preheat oven to 350°F.

2 In a large, heavy pot, heat oil and cook onion and garlic until just soft, about 3 minutes.

3 Add remaining sauce ingredients and bring to a boil. Simmer for 10 minutes. For a smoother sauce, mash tomatoes during simmering.

4 Steam spinach for 3 to 4 minutes; drain, cool, and squeeze excess water from spinach.

5 In a large bowl, mix filling ingredients with a fork. To assemble, stuff each cooked shell with about 2 T of the filling.

6 Spread ½ cup of the sauce in the bottoms of two 13 × 9-inch baking dishes. Arrange stuffed shells in a single layer. Pour remainder of sauce over shells.

7 Cover with aluminum foil and bake at 350°F for 24 to 30 minutes. To serve: Arrange four stuffed shells on a plate and cover with sauce. *Note:* This dish freezes well.

Nutrition Information Per Serving	
Calories 225	Protein (g). 16.5
Fat (g) 5.5	Sodium (mg) 1200
Fiber (g). 2.5	Carbohydrates (g) 30
	Cholesterol (mg). . . . . >1

Mediterranean Artichoke Hearts and White Bean Stew

—Amanda Cushman

Serves 8

1 Place artichokes in cold water with the lemon juice. Heat the olive oil in a large saucepan and add scallions, garlic, and red pepper, and sauté 3 minutes. Add drained artichokes, ¼ cup of the chicken broth, and salt and pepper. Cover and cook over low heat about 30 minutes, until artichokes are tender.

2 Add beans, remaining broth, tomatoes, zucchini, thyme, and basil, and cover. Cook another 15 minutes.

3 Add salt and pepper to taste, and serve.

Nutrition Information Per Serving

Calories	275	Protein (g)	17
Fat (g)	4.5	Sodium (mg)	165
Fiber (g)	13	Carbohydrates (g)	50
		Cholesterol (mg)	0

8 artichokes, trimmed, choke removed, hearts sliced

Juice of 1 lemon

2 T olive oil

2 bunches scallions, trimmed, sliced in 1-inch lengths

5 garlic cloves, sliced

1 red bell pepper, seeded and diced

1 cup low-fat chicken broth

Salt and pepper

One 16-oz can white beans, rinsed and drained

6 plum tomatoes, peeled, seeded, and chopped

1 zucchini, halved lengthwise and diced

2 tsp chopped thyme

2 T chopped basil

Chickpea Salad with Olives and Basil

Serves 8

Two 15-oz cans chickpeas, rinsed
  and drained

4 ripe tomatoes, halved, seeded,
  and chopped

2 celery stalks, diced

3 scallions, thinly sliced

½ cup Kalamata olives, pitted
  and chopped

8 basil leaves, julienned

½ cup chopped parsley

2 T olive oil

Juice of 2 lemons

3 T capers

Salt and pepper

—Amanda Cushman

Combine the chickpeas in a large bowl with remaining ingredients; toss and serve. Can be made a day ahead.

Nutrition Information Per Serving	
Calories 230	Protein (g) 7
Fat (g) 8.5	Sodium (mg) 465
Fiber (g) 6	Carbohydrates (g) 35
	Cholesterol (mg) 0

Mediterranean Tabouleh Salad
with Parsley and Mint

—Amanda Cushman

Serves 6

1 Combine the tabouleh and water in a small saucepan and season with salt. Bring to a boil, cover, remove from heat, and let sit for 15 minutes. Uncover and allow to cool.

2 Combine the remaining ingredients in a large serving bowl and toss well. Add tabouleh and toss. Taste for seasoning.

1 cup tabouleh (bulgur wheat), medium grain, rinsed and drained

1 ½ cups cold water

Salt

1 ½ cups chopped Italian (flat-leaf) parsley

4 ripe tomatoes, chopped

1 bunch scallions, minced

⅓ cup chopped mint leaves

3 stalks celery, finely diced

3 T olive oil

6 T lemon juice

Salt and pepper

Nutrition Information Per Serving

Calories	160	Protein (g)	3
Fat (g)	5	Sodium (mg)	120
Fiber (g)	2.5	Carbohydrates (g)	15
		Cholesterol (mg)	6

Goat Cheese and Black Olive Timbales with Baby Greens

—Frances Trzeciak

Vinaigrette:

1 T French mustard (such as Dijon)

1 garlic clove, minced

¼ cup extra-virgin olive oil

Salt and pepper

12 oz goat cheese (such as Montrachet)

3 large eggs

¾ cup finely chopped Kalamata olives (or any marinated black olives)

Butter

¾ lb baby greens (mesclun mix)

Fresh chopped chives, for garnish

1 Prepare vinaigrette. Salt and pepper to taste. Set aside.

2 Preheat oven to 350°F. Crumble goat cheese with a fork. In food processor, process the cheese with the eggs to a smooth texture. Add chopped olives and blend well.

3 Divide mixture between six buttered medium-size ramekins. (Make sure the bottom of each ramekin is well buttered.) Set the ramekins in baking pan with hot water; the water should come halfway up the sides of the ramekins.

4 Bake for 25 minutes. For a more golden color, finish them under the broiler, if you wish. Remove from hot water and set aside to cool.

5 Toss greens with vinaigrette, arrange on plates, and invert one ramekin on each. Garnish with chives.

Nutrition Information Per Serving

Calories	450	Protein (g)	20
Fat (g)	39	Sodium (mg)	430
Fiber (g)	>1	Carbohydrates (g)	5
		Cholesterol (mg)	150

Greek *Chorta*

—Nikki Rose

Serves 8

4 pounds of raw greens; allow at
least ½ lb of raw greens per
person
½ cup olive oil
2 small garlic cloves, finely
chopped
Juice of 1 lemon
Salt and pepper, to taste

The traditional Greek *chorta* is a combination of greens that grow wild on the hillsides and are handpicked by villagers. A typical *chorta* combination includes mustard greens, arugula, dandelion greens, beet greens, curly endive, sorrel, kale, collards, and purslane (which isn't available in North American markets, but which you might find in your garden), depending on availability. Boiled or steamed, seasoned with olive oil, lemon or vinegar, salt and pepper, and served cold or at room temperature, *chorta* is typically drained of its cooking juices, which also contain the golden vitamins. Greeks often reserve this juice to drink later, as a nutritional beverage.

1 Rinse greens thoroughly and remove tough stems. (A water-saving technique is to fill a clean sink or basin with 6 inches of fresh cold water; add trimmed greens, and submerge to allow sand to fall to the bottom of the sink. You may want to repeat once.) Transfer greens in small quantities to a colander and rinse again until greens are completely clean.

2 In a large, heavy, stainless steel or nonstick stockpot (not aluminum), over medium-high heat, add olive oil and heat for 30 seconds.

3 Add minced garlic and sauté 30 seconds more (avoid browning the garlic; it will be bitter).

4 Add greens that take the longest to cook, such as kale and collards. Simmer for 30 minutes, stirring occasionally with a wooden spoon. A good rule of thumb: The tougher the raw greens, the longer the cooking time. Beet greens should be cooked separately and combined at the last minute, as their intense color may turn the mixture brown.

5 Add more delicate greens, such as arugula or spinach, and simmer just until wilted.

6 Serve in a bowl with 1 to 2 T cooking juice; splash with lemon and olive oil. Season with salt and pepper, to taste.

Note: Adding salt or acid (lemon or vinegar) during cooking will turn certain brilliantly green vegetables into an unappetizing muted green. To be safe, add salt at serving time.

Greek Chorta (cont.)

Nutrition Information Per Serving

Calories	170	Protein (g)	4
Fat (g)	14	Sodium (mg)	45
Fiber (g)	2.5	Carbohydrates (g)	10
		Cholesterol (mg)	0

White Onion Pizza

—Maxine Clark

This succulent golden pizza is the forerunner of the French *pissaladière*. The onions are cooked in olive oil to a creamy softness, then spread onto the pizza dough before baking. Add more herbs if you like—dried herbs work well. If you hate anchovies, leave them out, but they do add a delicious savory saltiness to the sweet onions!

1 To make the pizza dough, mix yeast and sugar in a medium bowl, then whisk in the warm water. Set aside for 10 minutes until frothy.

2 Sift the flour into a large bowl and make a well in the center. Pour in the yeast mixture, olive oil, and salt. Mix together with a wooden spoon, then use hands until the dough comes together.

3 With clean, dry hands, knead the dough on a floured surface for 10 minutes until smooth and elastic. If too soft to handle, knead in a little more flour. Place in a clean oiled bowl and cover with a damp tea towel. Let rise for about 1 hour until doubled in size.

4 Meanwhile, peel and finely slice the onions.

5 Heat the oil in a heavy-based saucepan. Add the onions and cook over a gentle heat, stirring occasionally for 40 minutes to 1 hour until they are completely soft and golden, although not brown. Stir in the chopped herbs.

6 Preheat the oven to 450°F. Roll out the dough into a 12-inch circle on a large, floured baking sheet.

7 Spoon the onions on top of the dough and spread evenly. Sprinkle dough with anchovy fillets and olives. Bake for 15 minutes until golden and crisp. Garnish with rosemary sprigs and oregano leaves. Serve immediately.

Variation: Cover the base with sliced mozzarella before spreading with the onions. Sprinkle with 2 T freshly grated Parmesan cheese.

Serves 4

Pizza dough:

½ oz (½ T) yeast

Pinch of sugar

1 cup warm water

1 ½ cups enriched white flour

2 T olive oil

½ tsp salt

Topping:

2 lbs white onions

⅓ cup olive oil

1 T chopped fresh oregano

1 T chopped fresh rosemary

12 anchovy fillets in oil, drained

16 black olives, pitted

Rosemary sprigs and oregano
   leaves for garnish

White Onion Pizza *(cont.)*

Nutrition Information Per Serving	
Calories 365	Protein (g) 7
Fat (g) 20	Sodium (mg) 580
Fiber (g) 2.5	Carbohydrates (g) 40
	Cholesterol (mg) 7

Pasta Alla Carrettiera (Carter's Pasta)

—Maxine Clark

Serves 6

1 Peel and chop the tomatoes, retaining all the juice, and transfer to a medium bowl.

2 In a food processor, process the garlic, basil, chili flakes, and a pinch of salt, adding the oil slowly until smooth. Add mixture to the chopped tomatoes.

3 Cook the spaghetti in boiling salted water until *al dente;* drain, reserving 2 T of the cooking water.

4 In a serving bowl, toss spaghetti with half the cheese and the cooking liquid, then mix in the tomato mixture.

5 Sprinkle with the remaining cheese.

6 ripe tomatoes

4 to 5 garlic cloves, peeled

1 cup fresh basil leaves

Pinch dried chili flakes

Salt

½ cup olive oil

1½ lbs dried spaghetti

1 cup part-skim salted ricotta or grated pecorino cheese

Extra cheese for garnish

Nutrition Information Per Serving	
Calories 675	Protein (g) 20.5
Fat (g) 23	Sodium (mg) 70
Fiber (g) 4.5	Carbohydrates (g) 95
	Cholesterol (mg) 15

Shrimp with Lobster Sauce

Serves 4
—Lan Tan

½ lb shrimp, shelled and
deveined

1 tsp low-sodium soy sauce

2 tsp rice wine

¾ tsp cornstarch

Seasoning sauce:

2 tsp low-sodium soy sauce

2 tsp rice wine

1 tsp oyster sauce

Pinch white pepper

¾ cup fat-free chicken broth

1 ½ tsp cornstarch mixed with
1 T water

1 ½ T vegetable oil

1 garlic clove, peeled and
coarsely chopped

1 tsp salted black beans, rinsed
and coarsely chopped

2 oz ground pork or chicken

1 egg, lightly beaten

1 stalk scallion, split in half and
cut into 1-inch pieces

2 cups cooked rice

1 Rinse shrimp under cold running water and pat dry with paper towel. Mix soy sauce, rice wine, and cornstarch. Add to shrimp and refrigerate for about 30 minutes.

2 Prepare the seasoning sauce. Set aside.

3 Dissolve cornstarch in water.

4 Heat I T oil in wok or Dutch oven. Add shrimp and stir-fry until they turn pink in color, about 2 minutes. Remove and set aside.

5 Heat ½ T oil in wok or Dutch oven. Add garlic and black beans. Stir-fry for a few seconds and then add ground meat. Continue stirring until meat separates and turns white, about I minute. Add the seasoning sauce.

6 Bring to a boil. Add cornstarch mixture and stir constantly until sauce thickens, about I minute. Add the cooked shrimp, beaten egg, and scallions. Stir gently for about 5 seconds. Serve with rice.

Nutrition Information Per Serving with ½ Cup Cooked White Rice	
Calories 290	Protein (g) 20
Fat (g) 8.5	Sodium (mg) 280
Fiber (g) . . . . >1	Carbohydrates (g) 30
	Cholesterol (mg) 145

Grilled Salmon with Sesame Teriyaki Glaze

—Francine Fielding

Serves 4

1 In a small bowl, combine soy sauce, mirin, sesame oil, brown sugar, garlic, ginger, and red pepper flakes. Whisk together.

2 Place salmon fillets in a shallow glass or ceramic dish. Pour half of the soy sauce mixture over the salmon. Turn the salmon to completely coat with the marinade. Cover with plastic wrap and refrigerate for 30 minutes. Reserve the remaining marinade.

3 Preheat grill.

4 Remove salmon from marinade and place on grill, skin side down. Grill on both sides, about 5 to 6 minutes per side, depending on thickness.

5 Meanwhile, place remaining marinade in small saucepan. Bring to a boil until marinade starts to thicken, about 2 to 3 minutes.

6 Pour sauce over cooked salmon fillets, then sprinkle with toasted sesame seeds. Serve with rice.

⅓ cup soy sauce

⅓ cup mirin (Japanese rice wine)

1 T sesame oil

1 T brown sugar

1 T finely minced ginger

1 T finely minced garlic

¼ tsp dried hot red pepper flakes

Four 4-oz salmon fillets, boned, skin on

1 T toasted sesame seeds

2 cups cooked rice

Nutrition Information Per Serving with ½ Cup Cooked White Rice

Calories	335	Protein (g)	24
Fat (g)	8	Sodium (mg)	870
Fiber (g)	1	Carbohydrates (g)	35
		Cholesterol (mg)	50

Japanese Grilled Yellowtail (or Swordfish)

Serves 4

—*Kiyoko Konishi*

Marinade:

2 T sugar

2 T low-sodium soy sauce

1 T rice wine

2 tsp sesame oil

Four 4-oz yellowtail tuna or
    swordfish fillets

Diced scallions for garnish

2 cups cooked rice

1 Prepare the marinade.

2 Place fish in a shallow glass or ceramic dish. Pour marinade over the fish. Marinate for 15 minutes, turning occasionally.

3 Preheat grill.

4 Remove fish from marinade; reserve marinade for later.

5 Grill fish on both sides until lightly browned, about 5 minutes per side, depending on thickness.

6 Meanwhile, place remaining marinade in small saucepan. Bring to a boil and boil for 2 minutes.

7 Place fish on serving dish. Pour marinade over fish. Top with scallions. Serve with rice.

Nutrition Information Per Serving	
Calories 145	Protein (g) 25
Fat (g) 5	Sodium (mg) 40
Fiber (g) 0	Carbohydrates (g) 0
	Cholesterol (mg) 0

Steamed Fish, Cantonese Style

—*Lan Tan*

Serves 4

1 Rinse fish in cold running water and pat dry with paper towel. Score fish crosswise on both sides at 1-inch intervals. Place the fish in a shallow bowl or heat-proof plate such as a Pyrex pie plate.

2 Combine soy sauce, rice wine, vegetable oil, and pepper in a small bowl and mix well. Pour over fish. Sprinkle scallions and ginger around fish.

3 Bring 1 to 2 inches of water to boil in a wok. Place plate in bamboo steamer basket, and place over boiling water in wok. Steam for about 12 minutes.

4 Remove the fish bowl and transfer the fish and sauce to a large platter. Serve immediately.

1 lb fresh fish (such as red snapper, salmon, sea bass, or sole)

1 ½ T low-sodium soy sauce

2 tsp rice wine

2 tsp vegetable oil

Pinch white pepper

3 stalks scallions, split in half and cut into 3-inch lengths

1 ½ T julienned fresh ginger

Nutrition Information Per Serving	
Calories 170	Protein (g) 25
Fat (g) 6	Sodium (mg) 305
Fiber (g) . . . . <1	Carbohydrates (g) 3
	Cholesterol (mg) 60

Shrimp with Mixed Vegetables

Serves 4

—Lan Tan

Marinade:

2 tsp low-sodium soy sauce

2 tsp rice wine

1 tsp cornstarch

1/2 tsp grated ginger

1/2 lb shrimp, shelled and
   deveined

4 dried black mushrooms

Sauce:

2 tsp fish sauce

2 tsp oyster sauce

1 tsp rice wine

1 tsp sesame oil

1/2 tsp sugar

2 tsp cornstarch with a pinch of
   pepper

3/4 cup low-sodium chicken broth

1 T vegetable oil

2 garlic cloves, coarsely chopped

3 cups bok choy, shredded or
   thinly sliced

1/2 cup thinly sliced onion

1/2 julienned red bell pepper

1 cup bean sprouts

1 T sautéed shallots (optional)

2 cups cooked rice

1 Prepare marinade. Add shrimp and marinate in refrigerator for about 30 minutes.

2 Soak mushrooms in hot water for about 20 minutes or until soft. Drain, remove and discard tough stems, and julienne mushroom caps.

3 Combine the sauce ingredients in a small bowl; set aside.

4 Heat 1/2 T oil in wok. Add shrimp and stir-fry for about 2 minutes or until shrimp turns white. Remove and set aside.

5 Heat 1/2 T oil in wok. Add garlic, bok choy, onion, mushrooms, and red bell pepper. Stir for about 2 minutes. Add the sauce. Bring to a boil and stir until thick, about 1 minute. Add bean sprouts and the cooked shrimp. Cook 1 to 2 minutes until heated through. Garnish with shallots if desired. Serve with rice.

Nutrition Information Per Serving with 1/2 Cup Cooked White Rice	
Calories 265	Protein (g). 17.5
Fat (g) 4	Sodium (mg) 290
Fiber (g). 2.5	Carbohydrates (g) 40
	Cholesterol (mg). 90

Provençal Sea Bass

—Lynn Kutner

1 Slice tomatoes about ¼-inch thick. Salt lightly and place on a wire rack to drain for 30 minutes. Dry on paper towels and set aside.

2 Chop the leek and sauté slowly in olive oil until tender (8 to 10 minutes). Set aside.

3 Chop garlic and cook slowly in 1 to 2 T olive oil until soft but not browned (3 to 5 minutes). Combine the garlic, parsley, and bread crumbs in a bowl. Season with freshly ground pepper.

4 Preheat oven to 375°F; place rack in upper third of oven.

5 Lightly oil a baking dish that you can serve from. Spread leeks in dish.

6 Lightly salt and pepper fish. Place on top of leeks.

7 Arrange chopped olives on top of fish.

8 Cover olives with ¾ of crumb mixture.

9 Arrange tomatoes on crumbs. Sprinkle with reserved crumbs. Drizzle with 1 T of olive oil and bake 20 to 25 minutes.

Serves 3

2 plum tomatoes

Salt and pepper

1 leek, well-washed (use white and tender light green parts)

2 garlic cloves

Olive oil

⅓ cup chopped fresh parsley

1 cup fresh bread crumbs

1 lb sea bass fillets, cut into serving pieces

8 to 10 Kalamata olives, pitted and chopped

Nutrition Information Per Serving	
Calories 290	Protein (g) 30
Fat (g) 12	Sodium (mg) 275
Fiber (g) 2	Carbohydrates (g) 15
	Cholesterol (mg) 60

Coriander-Crusted Tuna with Parsley Dressing

Serves 4

¼ cup coriander seeds

1 tsp salt

½ tsp black pepper

Four 5-oz tuna steaks, about 1 ½
  inches thick

2 egg whites, lightly whisked

1 T olive oil

Parsley dressing (see recipe on
  page 205)

2 T chopped parsley

—Amanda Cushman

1 Heat oven to 350°F.

2 Crack the coriander seeds with the bottom of a heavy skillet, or grind them in a pepper mill. Mix in a plate with the salt and pepper.

3 Brush the tuna with the egg whites, and press spice mixture onto each piece of tuna.

4 In a large skillet, heat the olive oil. Sear the tuna for 1 minute on each side. Place the pan in the oven and heat the fish for 3 minutes.

5 Remove from oven and slice the fish into ¼-inch slices. Divide among 4 plates and arrange in overlapping slices. Drizzle with the parsley dressing and garnish with the chopped parsley.

Nutrition Information Per Serving	
Calories 285	Protein (g) 40
Fat (g) 12	Sodium (mg) 625
Fiber (g) . . . . >1	Carbohydrates (g) . . . . >1
	Cholesterol (mg) 65

Parsley Dressing

—Amanda Cushman

Makes 1 cup

1 Cook orange juice in a small saucepan over medium heat until reduced to ¼ cup, about 12 minutes. Cool.

2 Toast the cumin seeds in a skillet until aromatic, about 4 minutes. Grind in a spice grinder.

3 In a food processor, blend the orange juice with the parsley until smooth. Add oil, cumin, and lemon juice, and mix well. Season with salt and cayenne pepper.

1 cup fresh orange or lemon juice

2 tsp cumin seeds

1 cup parsley leaves

½ cup canola oil

1 T lemon juice (if using lemon juice above, omit this juice)

Salt and cayenne pepper, to taste

Nutrition Information Per Tablespoon

Calories 75	Protein (g) . . . . >1
Fat (g) 7	Sodium (mg) 17
Fiber (g) . . . . >1	Carbohydrates (g) 3.5
	Cholesterol (mg) 0

Seafood Soup with Rouille

Serves 4

—Francis Trzeciak

Rouille:

1 garlic clove

½ cup olive oil

1 tsp paprika

Salt and cayenne pepper, to

    taste

1 potato, peeled and boiled

Soup:

8 sea scallops

¼ lb red snapper fillet

¼ lb monkfish

12 mussels

4 large shrimp

1 cup dry white wine

3 T grated fresh ginger

Fresh thyme

1 pinch saffron

Salt and cayenne pepper, to

    taste

½ garlic clove, minced

1 small leek, julienned

4 toasted baguette slices for

    garnish

1 In food processor, make rouille: Process garlic, then add olive oil, paprika, salt, cayenne, and potato. Process until smooth. Refrigerate until ready to use.

2 Cut scallops, red snapper, monkfish, and mussels into small cubes. Peel and devein shrimp. Do not discard shells.

3 Over high heat, boil wine, 1 cup water, ginger, thyme, saffron, salt, and cayenne pepper. Add shrimp shells. Boil for 5 minutes until liquid is reduced and is a nice deep yellow color. Strain stock in fine sieve. Return to same pan. Add fish, and garlic. Cook for 1 to 2 minutes. Set aside and cover with a lid.

4 Divide seafood by 4 and arrange in deep soup bowls with broth and julienne of leeks for garnish.

5 Spread the rouille on baguette rounds and top each bowl with a rouille crouton.

Nutrition Information Per Serving			
Calories	765	Protein (g)	75
Fat (g)	25	Sodium (mg)	1525
Fiber (g)	2	Carbohydrates (g)	45
		Cholesterol (mg)	170

Paupiette of Sea Bass with Tapenade and Sauce Provençale in Thin Potato Crust

—*Francis Trzeciak*

Serves 4

1 Sprinkle fillets with salt, pepper, and fresh thyme. Spread the black olive puree on each fillet. Cut each potato lengthwise into long, thin slices with a vegetable slicer or mandoline (about 16 slices per potato; you will need 8 slices per fillet). *Note:* Do not rinse potatoes.

2 Place the first potato slice perpendicular to the fillet, starting on the left side. Place the second slice overlapping the first one. Continue in this manner until the fillet is covered.

3 Gently lift each fillet with a spatula, folding the ends of the potatoes underneath. Place finished fillets to one side (can be made up to 1 hour in advance).

4 Turn oven to 425°F. Heat the oil in a sauté or nonstick pan over high heat. When oil is hot, sauté *paupiettes* until golden brown (1 to 2 minutes per side). Remove from pan. Place in a baking pan and finish cooking in the oven for 5 minutes.

To make *Sauce Provençale:*

1 Discard oil from pan used to sauté *paupiettes.* Return pan to stove and add 1 T olive oil, shallots, and garlic. Add yellow and red peppers; stir and continue to sauté.

2 Add wine; reduce heat and simmer. When mixture is reduced by half, add 1 tsp butter and fresh thyme.

To serve:

Remove fish from oven. Pour sauce onto each plate. Place one fillet on top of sauce in middle of plate. Garnish with thyme leaves if desired.

Ingredients

Four 5-oz sea bass fillets
 (skinless and boneless)
Salt
Freshly ground pepper
3 sprigs fresh thyme
2 tsp black olive puree
2 large baking potatoes, peeled

Sauce Provençale:

1 T extra-virgin olive oil
3 shallots, chopped
3 medium garlic cloves, chopped
1 yellow bell pepper, diced
1 red bell pepper, diced
1 cup dry white wine
1 tsp unsalted butter
Fresh thyme

Nutrition Information Per Serving			
Calories	290	Protein (g)	30
Fat (g)	7.5	Sodium (mg)	120
Fiber (g)	1.5	Carbohydrates (g)	20
		Cholesterol (mg)	60

Swedish Shrimp Salad

Serves 4

— Birgitta Rasmusson

1 lb fresh cooked shrimp

8 fresh mushrooms

1 head lettuce

1 tomato

8 asparagus spears, cut in ¼-
    inch pieces

1 cup frozen peas, thawed

Dressing:

2 T red wine vinegar

2 T canola or olive oil

Salt and pepper, to taste

1 Peel the shrimp, slice the mushrooms, shred the lettuce, and cut tomato into thin wedges.

2 Mix these ingredients with asparagus and peas, and toss with dressing. Season with salt and pepper. (*Note:* Swedes traditionally serve the salad with toast as a first course or as a luncheon or supper dish.)

Nutrition Information Per Serving	
Calories 220	Protein (g) 22
Fat (g) 8.5	Sodium (mg) 245
Fiber (g) 5	Carbohydrates (g) 15
	Cholesterol (mg) 165

Shrimp with Feta Cheese and Tomatoes

—Nikki Rose

Serves 6

1 Preheat oven to 400°F. Coat a 9 × 10-inch heavy baking dish with 1 tsp olive oil.

2 In a heavy sauté pan over medium heat, add 2 T of olive oil, then the onions, and sauté until tender. Add garlic and sauté 1 minute more.

3 Reduce heat and add tomatoes, white wine, and parsley, 2 T oregano, and the pepper. Simmer for 15 minutes to create a light sauce.

4 Meanwhile, in another sauté pan over medium-high heat, add 3 T olive oil, then the shrimp, and sauté just 1 minute.

5 Transfer shrimp to the baking dish; top with tomato sauce, the remaining oregano, then the crumbled feta.

6 Cover and bake 10 to 15 minutes, just until flavors meld—no longer or the shrimp will be tough. Serve at once as an appetizer with crispy bread on the side, or as a main dish over bow-tie pasta.

Variation: For added heat, add a small pinch of Tabasco sauce or dried pepper flakes when sautéing the shrimp. For best flavor, avoid substituting dried oregano for fresh. Also, feta cheese can be salty, so add extra salt with caution.

Ingredients

5 T olive oil

1 large onion, halved and thinly sliced

2 garlic cloves, minced

2 lbs tomatoes, peeled, seeded, and chopped

1 cup dry white wine

3 T finely chopped fresh parsley

1/4 cup finely chopped fresh oregano leaves

Freshly ground black pepper, to taste

2 lbs large shrimp, peeled and deveined

3/4 lb good quality feta cheese, crumbled

Nutrition Information Per Serving

Calories	485	Protein (g)	40
Fat (g)	25	Sodium (mg)	875
Fiber (g)	2.5	Carbohydrates (g)	15
		Cholesterol (mg)	280

Pesce al Sale (Salt-Baked Fish)

—*Maxine Clark*

2 to 4 lbs whole large firm-fleshed fish, such as red snapper or trout, neither gutted nor scaled

2 lbs (at least) sea salt or Kosher salt

1 egg white

3 T water

This excellent method of cooking conserves the juices without in any way oversalting the flesh. The quantity of salt is rather daunting unless you have your own salt flats just down the road!

1 Rinse fish under cold running water, but do not scale or gut. Pat dry.

2 Pour enough salt into an oblong baking dish to make a 1-inch layer.

3 Mix the egg white with the water and sprinkle half the liquid over the salt. Lay the fish on the salt bed, and pour enough salt around and over it to cover it completely.

4 Sprinkle with the remaining egg white and water. Bake in the oven at 375°F for about 1 hour, the temperature adjusted up or down depending on the size of the fish.

5 Place the fish, still encased in its snowy armor, in the middle of the table. Crack open the salt crust with a hammer. A little theatricality is quite proper! The skin will come off with the salt, revealing perfectly cooked, succulent flesh without a trace of saltiness.

Nutrition Information Per Serving			
Calories	305	Protein (g)	60
Fat (g)	4	Sodium (mg)	205
Fiber (g)	>1	Carbohydrates (g)	>1
		Cholesterol (mg)	110

Polpette di Tonno (Tuna Patties)

—Maxine Clark

Serves 6

Palermo cooks prepare this dish with sardines instead of tuna; if neither fresh sardines nor fresh tuna is available, fresh mackerel fillets will do.

1. Bone and skin the fish and chop it into very small pieces.

2. Soak bread crumbs in milk for 10 minutes or until soft. Squeeze out excess liquid and mix the crumbs with the fish. Add currants, pine nuts, parsley, cheese, salt, pepper, and egg. Work these ingredients together well with your hands or mixer until they are thoroughly combined, then shape them into small patties about 2 inches in diameter.

3. Dip the patties in flour and brown them on both sides in a few tablespoons of olive oil. Pour tomato sauce over the patties and simmer them for 10 to 15 minutes.

1 lb fresh tuna or 1½ lbs fresh sardines

1 cup dry white bread crumbs

½ cup skim milk

2 T currants, plumped in hot water for 5 minutes

2 T pine nuts

1 T chopped fresh parsley

2 T grated Pecorino cheese

Salt and freshly ground black pepper

1 egg, beaten

Flour

Olive oil

2 cups tomato sauce (such as your favorite ready-made brand)

Nutrition Information Per Serving	
Calories 255	Protein (g) 25
Fat (g) 7.5	Sodium (mg) 740
Fiber (g) 2.5	Carbohydrates (g) 20
	Cholesterol (mg) 60

Char-Grilled Squid with Chilies and Eggplant

Serves 4

—Maxine Clark

1½ lbs baby squid, or large ones
    with pouches sliced into
    rings before cooking

2 garlic cloves

2 small red chili peppers

4 T olive oil

Juice of 1 lemon

1 tsp chili sauce

2 medium eggplant

Salt

Vegetable oil, for basting

Arugula

Lemon wedges

Baby squid are marinated in chili, garlic, and olive oil, then char-grilled to a smoky sweetness and served on a bed of arugula and grilled eggplant, which soak up the spicy juices and cut through the richness. For best results, use a searing-hot griddle or a grill at its highest setting.

1 To prepare the squid, rinse well. Hold the body in one hand and firmly pull the tentacles with the other hand, to remove the soft contents of the body pouch. Cut the tentacles just in front of the eyes and discard the body contents; reserve the tentacles. Rinse the body pouches under cold running water.

2 Peel and finely chop the garlic; halve, remove seeds, and chop the chilies. Place in a shallow dish with the olive oil, lemon juice, and chili sauce.

3 Add the squid pouches and tentacles; stir well; cover and marinate in refrigerator for 2 hours.

4 Meanwhile, slice the eggplant into thin slices. Spread eggplant slices in a colander and sprinkle with salt. Set aside for 20 minutes. Rinse well and pat dry with paper towels.

5 Heat a griddle until smoking and brush with oil. (Alternatively, preheat the grill to high and brush the eggplant slices with oil.) Cook eggplant slices in batches for 2 minutes on each side. Keep warm in a warm oven.

6 Remove the squid from the marinade using a slotted spoon, reserving the marinade. Heat the griddle once more and cook (or grill) squid pouches for 2 minutes on each side. Transfer the squid pouches to a warmed dish; keep hot.

7 Add the squid tentacles to the griddle (or grill) and cook for 1 to 2 minutes. Pour the marinade into a pan and heat gently. Arrange the eggplant slices on warmed serving plates. Top each with a bed of arugula. Pile the squid on top and spoon over a little marinade. Serve with lemon wedges.

Char-Grilled Squid with Chilies and Eggplant *(cont.)*

Nutrition Information Per Serving

Calories 340	Protein (g) 30
Fat (g) 16	Sodium (mg) 80
Fiber (g) 5	Carbohydrates (g) 20
	Cholesterol (mg) 400

Scandinavian Fish Soup

Serves 4

—Birgitta Rasmusson

1 T margarine or butter

2 carrots, thinly sliced

1 leek, thinly sliced

1½ T Flour

4 cups fish stock

1 bay leaf

1 lb fish fillets, thinly sliced

⅔ cup frozen peas

Salt and white pepper, to taste

Chopped dill or parsley for
  garnish

1 In a saucepan, melt margarine or butter. Add the carrots and leek and cook for a few minutes. Sprinkle with flour. Add the fish stock and bay leaf. Cover and let simmer for 10 minutes.

2 Add the fish fillet slices and simmer a few minutes more. Add the peas. Season with salt and pepper to taste. Garnish each serving with dill or parsley.

Nutrition Information Per Serving			
Calories	270	Protein (g)	23
Fat (g)	9.5	Sodium (mg)	365
Fiber (g)	3	Carbohydrates (g)	15
		Cholesterol (mg)	70

Smoked Salmon Omelette with Potatoes

—Birgitta Rasmusson

Serves 4

1 Sauté the potatoes in oil over medium heat for several minutes until tender. Add salmon slices.

2 Mix eggs with water, salt, pepper, and dill. Pour the mixture over potatoes and salmon, and reduce heat. Cook omelette over low heat until eggs are set.

3 Garnish with chives. Serve with sliced tomatoes and bread.

4 to 6 potatoes, boiled, cooled, and diced into small cubes

1 T vegetable oil

6 oz smoked salmon, thinly sliced

6 eggs

1/3 cup water

Salt and pepper

1 T chopped dill

2 T chopped chives

Nutrition Information Per Serving	
Calories 390	Protein (g) 21.5
Fat (g) 12	Sodium (mg) 430
Fiber (g) 4.5	Carbohydrates (g) 50
	Cholesterol (mg) 285

Fillet of Flounder with Capers and Beets

Serves 4

Four 6-oz flounder fillets, fresh or
    frozen

2 T flour

2 T fine dry bread crumbs

2 tsp salt

1 egg white, lightly beaten

2 T butter or margarine

Garnish:

2 T capers

3 T finely chopped pickled beets

1 T finely chopped parsley

—Birgitta Rasmusson

1 If using frozen flounder, thaw thoroughly.

2 Mix flour, bread crumbs, and salt.

3 Dip fillets in beaten egg white, then coat with bread crumb mixture.

4 In medium skillet, melt I T of the butter. Add the fish and cook until golden brown. Remove to a warm platter.

5 Brown the remaining butter or margarine; stir in the capers, beets, and parsley. Pour over the fish. Serve with boiled potatoes.

Nutrition Information Per Serving	
Calories 205	Protein (g) 27.5
Fat (g) 6.8	Sodium (mg) 1330
Fiber (g) . . . . >1	Carbohydrates (g) 7.5
	Cholesterol (mg) 15

Sarde alla Beccaficu (Stuffed Sardines)

—Maxine Clark

Serves 4

Fresh sardines are easily boned with the flick of a finger. Here they are opened out and stuffed with a sweet and savory mixture of pine nuts, parsley, and raisins, then rolled and baked until tender. A tomato and onion salad is the perfect accompaniment.

1 Preheat the oven to 350°F. Scrape the scales from the sardines if necessary, then cut off the heads. Slit open the bellies and rinse the insides under cold running water. Lay, flesh-side down, on a board. Slide your thumb along the backbone, pressing firmly to release the flesh along its length. Take hold of the backbone at the head end and lift it out; the fish should now be open like a book.

2 In a small bowl, mix together the pine nuts, raisins, parsley, orange rind, salt, and pepper. Place a spoonful of stuffing on the flesh side of each fish. Roll up from the head end and secure with a toothpick if necessary.

3 Place the stuffed sardines into a small, greased ovenproof dish. It is important that the sardines are tightly packed together. Tuck in a few bay leaves here and there. Pour over the orange juice and olive oil. Season with salt and pepper, and bake for about 10 minutes. Serve hot or cold.

16 fresh sardines

¼ cup pine nuts, toasted

¼ cup raisins

3 T chopped fresh parsley

Finely grated orange rind

Salt and pepper

Bay leaves

Juice of 1 orange

⅓ cup olive oil

Nutrition Information Per Serving	
Calories 260	Protein (g) 13
Fat (g) 19	Sodium (mg) 230
Fiber (g) . . . . >1	Carbohydrates (g) 10
	Cholesterol (mg) 65

Ginger Pork

Serves 4

—Kiyoko Konishi

2 T low-sodium soy sauce

1 T rice wine

1 tsp sugar

8 oz pork loin, cut into thin strips

Vegetable oil

1½ T minced fresh ginger

1 large onion, cut into ½-inch chunks

2 cabbage leaves, shredded (1 cup)

1 medium red bell pepper, cut into ¼-inch strips (1 cup)

1 medium green bell pepper, cut into ¼-inch strips (1 cup)

1 In a small bowl, combine soy sauce, rice wine, and sugar. Add sliced pork and toss well. Cover with plastic wrap and refrigerate for 30 minutes.

2 In wok or large nonstick skillet, heat 1 T oil over high heat until hot, but not smoking.

3 Add 1 T ginger and stir-fry until fragrant, about 10 seconds. Add pork and cook until meat turns brown, about 2 minutes.

4 Remove pork and set aside.

5 Heat 1 T oil in wok and add ½ T ginger and the onions. Stir-fry until onions are tender, about 4 minutes.

6 Add cabbage and red and green bell peppers and cook until vegetables are tender, about 2 to 3 minutes.

7 Return pork to wok and cook until heated through, about 1 minute. Serve with steamed rice.

Nutrition Information Per Serving with ½ Cup Cooked White Rice

Calories	280	Protein (g)	13
Fat (g)	10	Sodium (mg)	30
Fiber (g)	2	Carbohydrates (g)	35
		Cholesterol (mg)	25

Rolled Beef with Vegetables

—Kiyoko Konishi

1 Place beef in freezer for about 30 minutes. Slice into 8 very thin slices. Set aside.

2 Blanch carrots and green beans until tender. Rinse under cold running water; drain and set aside.

3 Combine sauce ingredients. Set aside.

4 Pat beef slices dry. Coat with cornstarch and shake off excess.

5 Place 2 to 3 carrot slices and 2 to 3 green beans diagonally across each beef slice. Roll tightly and secure with a toothpick. Continue with remaining beef and vegetables.

6 In a large nonstick skillet, heat oil over medium-high heat until hot but not smoking. Add beef rolls, seam-side down. Cook until bottom is browned, then gently turn rolls and brown on all sides.

7 Add sauce to skillet. Turn heat to low and continue to cook rolls 4 more minutes. Remove from heat. Let rolls sit 3 to 4 minutes, then cut each in half.

8 Drizzle rolls with pan juices. Serve with mixed greens.

10 oz beef sirloin or tenderloin (approximately 6 inches long and 4 inches wide)

2 to 3 carrots, peeled and cut into strips 6 inches long by ¼ inch wide

8 oz green beans, trimmed, 6 inches long

Sauce:

½ cup water

2 T low-sodium soy sauce

1 T rice wine

1 T mirin

1 T sugar

Cornstarch

1 T vegetable oil

Nutrition Information Per Serving	
Calories 180	Protein (g) 12
Fat (g) 9.5	Sodium (mg) 345
Fiber (g) 2.5	Carbohydrates (g) 10
	Cholesterol (mg) 35

Japanese-Style Braised Beef and Potatoes

Serves 4

—Kiyoko Konishi

8 oz beef tenderloin or sirloin

1 T low-sodium soy sauce

2 tsp sake or dry sherry

2 large potatoes

1½ T vegetable oil

1 T grated ginger

2 onions, each cut into 8 wedges

2 carrots, cut into ⅛-inch rounds
   (½ cup)

1 cup water

¼ cup sake

2 T sugar

¼ cup low-sodium soy sauce

1 cup fresh or frozen (thawed)
   green peas, steamed for 1 to
   2 minutes

1 Cut beef into thin 2-inch-long strips.

2 In a small bowl, combine 1 T soy sauce and 2 tsp sake. Add beef and toss well. Cover with plastic wrap and refrigerate for 10 minutes.

3 Peel potatoes and cut each into 8 wedges. Soak in cold water for 5 minutes; drain.

4 In large nonstick skillet or wok, heat ½ T oil over high heat until hot but not smoking. Add beef and ginger and stir-fry until meat turns brown, about 2 minutes. Remove and set aside.

5 Add remaining oil to skillet. When heated, add onions and stir-fry for 3 to 4 minutes. Add potatoes and carrots, and mix well.

6 Add water, sake, and sugar, and cook, covered, until potatoes are almost tender, about 8 minutes. Add soy sauce and simmer until vegetables are tender, about 4 to 5 minutes longer.

7 Add green peas and cook 1 minute more until peas are heated through.

Nutrition Information Per Serving			
Calories	365	Protein (g)	17.5
Fat (g)	9.5	Sodium (mg)	800
Fiber (g)	6.5	Carbohydrates (g)	50
		Cholesterol (mg)	35

Sukiyaki Stir-Fry

—Francine Fielding

1 Place beef in freezer for 30 minutes. Remove and cut into very thin slices.

2 Cook the *shirataki* in boiling water for 2 minutes. Drain. Rinse under cold running water. Cut into bite-size pieces.

3 In small bowl, combine the dashi, mirin, soy sauce, and sugar. Mix well to dissolve the sugar. Set aside.

4 In a wok or large nonstick skillet, heat the vegetable oil over medium-high heat until hot but not smoking.

5 Add the ginger and beef, and cook until beef turns brown, about 2 minutes. Remove from the wok and set aside.

6 Heat the remaining T of oil in the wok over medium-high heat until hot but not smoking. Add the onion and scallions and stir-fry until onion starts to soften, about 3 minutes.

7 Add the shiitake and enoki mushrooms and cook 1 minute.

8 Add the *shirataki* and the dashi mixture. Bring mixture to a simmer. Add the spinach and cook until it wilts, about 1 minute.

9 Add cornstarch mixture and simmer, stirring constantly until sauce thickens, about 1 minute.

½ lb beef tenderloin

7-oz package *shirataki,* or 4 oz Chinese bean thread noodles

2 T dashi

2 T mirin

2 T low-sodium soy sauce

1 ½ tsp sugar

2 T vegetable oil

1 tsp finely minced ginger

1 cup thinly sliced onion

6 scallions, cut into ½-inch slices

8 fresh shiitake mushrooms, cut into quarters

4-oz package of enoki mushrooms, bottom 2 to 3 inches cut off

1 bunch fresh spinach, tough stems removed, cut in half crosswise

1 tsp cornstarch mixed with 1 T water

Nutrition Information Per Serving with ½ Cup Cooked White Rice	
Calories 525	Protein (g) 20
Fat (g) 20	Sodium (mg) 1160
Fiber (g). 4.5	Carbohydrates (g) 65
	Cholesterol (mg). 40

Tonkatsu

Serves 4

—Francine Fielding

10 oz boneless pork loin or
 tenderloin

Salt and pepper

¼ cup flour

1 large egg, beaten with 1 tsp
 water

1 cup dried bread crumbs

4 T ketchup

2 T Worcestershire sauce

1 T low-sodium soy sauce

2 to 3 T vegetable oil

4 cups shredded cabbage,
 soaked in cold water for 5
 minutes

Lemon wedges

1 Slice the pork on the diagonal into 12 thin slices.

2 Place the pork between two sheets of plastic wrap and gently pound with a mallet until about ⅛-inch thick.

3 Season the pork slices with salt and pepper.

4 Dredge the pork in the flour, shaking off the excess.

5 Dip each piece into the egg, then into the bread crumbs.

6 Place on a plate. Cover with plastic wrap and refrigerate for 30 minutes.

7 In a small bowl, combine the ketchup, Worcestershire sauce, and soy sauce, and set aside.

8 In a large nonstick skillet, heat 2 T oil until hot but not smoking.

9 Add the pork and cook until golden brown, about 1 to 2 minutes. Turn and cook the other side until golden brown and cooked through, about 1 minute more. Cook in 2 batches if necessary, using the additional T of oil.

10 On each plate, place 1 cup of the shredded cabbage and top with three slices of meat. Serve with ketchup mixture and lemon wedges.

Nutrition Information Per Serving with ½ Cup Cooked White Rice	
Calories 465	Protein (g) 25
Fat (g) 12.5	Sodium (mg) 655
Fiber (g) 4	Carbohydrates (g) 60
	Cholesterol (mg). 90

Mediterranean Roast Leg of Lamb

—Lynn Kutner

Serves 8

1 Mix all marinade ingredients to form a paste; brush or spoon over the lamb. Marinate from ½ hour to overnight. If you keep it overnight, refrigerate in a glass or stainless steel bowl covered with plastic.

2 When ready to cook, preheat oven to 450°F, with rack set in the middle of the oven. Place leg of lamb on V-shaped rack in a roasting pan. Roast at 450°F for 20 minutes. Then turn heat to 350°F and roast for 30 minutes; turn the leg over and roast for an additional 40 to 45 minutes. Lamb will be medium-rare (meat thermometer should read 145°F). If you like it rare, roast it for only 1 hour after turning down the heat.

Marinade:

4 to 6 garlic cloves, pressed

3 to 4 T *herbes de Provence* (or snipped fresh rosemary, basil, oregano, and thyme)

3 to 4 T Dijon mustard

3 to 4 T low-sodium soy sauce (for color)

3 to 5 T olive oil

7- to 8-pound leg of lamb, trimmed

Nutrition Information Per 4-oz Serving

Calories 205	Protein (g) 16
Fat (g) 15	Sodium (mg) 50
Fiber (g) . . . . >1	Carbohydrates (g) 0
	Cholesterol (mg) 60

Swedish Hash

Serves 4

—*Birgitta Rasmusson*

2 T butter or margarine

8 boiled potatoes, peeled and
   cut into small cubes

2 onions, finely chopped

3 oz smoked ham, cut into small
   cubes

1¾ cups boiled or roast beef, cut
   in small cubes

1 tsp salt

White pepper

Finely chopped fresh parsley

1 In medium skillet, melt half the butter. Add potato cubes and cook over medium heat until golden brown and tender. Transfer to a platter.

2 Add remaining butter or margarine to skillet, and cook onions until soft and translucent. Remove and mix with the potatoes.

3 Sauté the ham. Add the beef and brown it lightly. Return the potatoes and onions to the skillet and mix well. Add salt and pepper to taste. Heat the hash thoroughly. Garnish with chopped parsley. Serve with ketchup and a side salad.

Nutrition Information Per Serving			
Calories	715	Protein (g)	32
Fat (g)	20	Sodium (mg)	675
Fiber (g)	10	Carbohydrates (g)	100
		Cholesterol (mg)	75

Scandinavian Pork Chops in Applesauce

—Birgitta Rasmusson

—Birgitta Rasmusson

Serves 4

1 In medium frying pan, sauté the garlic, leek, and apple cubes in 1 tsp of the vegetable oil until apples are tender. Transfer mixture to a plate and set aside.

2 Add remaining vegetable oil to the pan, and sauté the pork chops until almost opaque. Season with salt and pepper.

3 Spread apple mixture over the chops; pour in apple juice. Let cook over medium heat for 10 minutes. Sprinkle with parsley, and serve with pasta or rice.

2 garlic cloves, finely chopped

1 leek, finely sliced

2 apples, peeled and diced

1 T vegetable oil

4 lean pork chops

 salt and pepper

¾ cup apple juice

2 T finely chopped parsley

Nutrition Information Per Serving	
Calories 170	Protein (g) 5.4
Fat (g) 9	Sodium (mg) 25
Fiber (g) 2	Carbohydrates (g) 20
	Cholesterol (mg) 20

Swedish Beef Patties with Onions

Serves 6

—Birgitta Rasmusson

2 cold boiled potatoes

1 lb lean ground beef

Salt and white pepper

$\frac{1}{3}$ cup water

2 T butter or margarine

2 large onions, sliced

1 Mash the potatoes and mix with the ground beef. Add salt, pepper, and water. Work the meat mixture until smooth and shape into patties.

2 Heat a skillet with I T butter. Add the onions and cook over moderate heat until golden brown. Transfer the onions to a platter and keep hot.

3 Melt the remaining butter in the skillet, and cook the patties over moderate heat until brown on both sides and cooked through. Serve patties with sautéed onions and vegetables of your choice.

Nutrition Information Per Serving			
Calories	300	Protein (g)	16
Fat (g)	16.9	Sodium (mg)	95
Fiber (g)	2.3	Carbohydrates (g)	20
		Cholesterol (mg)	60

Chicken and Beef Benachin

—Hope Farrell

Serves 6

1 Cut the chicken legs into thighs and drumsticks. Cut tip sirloin into ¾-inch cubes. Salt and pepper meats to taste. Heat 2 T peanut oil in a large, heavy pot or Dutch oven over medium-high heat, and brown the chicken pieces on all sides. Remove from pot and set aside. Add beef and brown on all sides; remove and set aside.

2 Lower heat to medium, add 1 T oil to pot and stir in onions. Sauté onions for 5 minutes. Add tomatoes, tomato paste, garlic, chili or pepper flakes, and bay leaves. Simmer for 5 minutes. Stir in chicken broth, and return chicken and beef to pot. Bring all to the simmer, and cook for 15 minutes.

3 Add cabbage, eggplant, and squash to the pot, bring back to the simmer, and cook, partially covered, for another 15 minutes, or until vegetables are tender.

4 While the vegetables are simmering, heat the remaining 1 T oil in another pot. Stir in the rice and green pepper and sauté for 5 minutes, stirring constantly. Set aside.

5 When the meats and vegetables are tender, taste for seasonings and add salt or pepper as necessary. Drain off 4 cups of liquid from the pot, and cover the pot to keep the meats and vegetables warm.

6 Stir the 4 cups of liquid into the rice. Bring to the simmer, cover, turn heat to low, and cook the rice for about 18 minutes, until tender and the liquid has been absorbed.

7 To serve, place the rice in a large oval serving dish. Arrange the chicken, beef, and vegetables attractively over the rice.

Ingredients

3 whole chicken legs (1 ½ lbs), skinned

½ lb boneless tip sirloin

Salt and pepper

4 T peanut oil, divided

4 large onions, sliced (1 ¼ lbs, 5 cups)

3 medium tomatoes, peeled and sliced (1 lb, 3 cups)

4 T tomato paste

4 large garlic cloves, minced (1 T)

One 3-inch hot chili pepper, seeded and minced, or ½ tsp red pepper flakes

2 bay leaves

4 cups nonfat chicken broth

½ small cabbage, cut along core into 6 wedges (¾ lb)

1 small eggplant, peeled and cut in 1-inch cubes (¾ lb, 3 cups)

1 small butternut squash, peeled, seeded, and cut in 1-inch cubes (½ lb, 1¾ cups)

2 cups long-grain white rice

1 large green bell pepper, seeded, de-ribbed, and cut into ½-inch squares (½ lb, 1⅓ cups)

Nutrition Information Per Serving

Calories	615	Protein (g)	30
Fat (g)	20	Sodium (mg)	300
Fiber (g)	7.5	Carbohydrates (g)	85
		Cholesterol (mg)	70

Pulla (Finnish Cardamom-Flavored Coffeebraid)

Makes 3 braids

—Beatrice Ojakangas

2 packages (2 T) active dry yeast

½ cup warm water (105°F to 115°F)

2 cups low-fat or skim milk, scalded and cooled to lukewarm

1 cup sugar

1 tsp salt

1 tsp freshly crushed cardamom seeds

4 large eggs, lightly beaten

8 to 9 cups unbleached all-purpose flour

½ cup (1 stick) butter, softened

Glaze and topping:

1 egg, beaten

½ cup sliced almonds

½ cup coarsely crushed sugar cubes

This moist, rich, lightly sweetened coffee bread is flavored with cardamom. For the best flavor, grind cardamom seeds just before adding them to the mixture. Cardamom that is already ground and packed in jars has lost its flavor.

1 In a large warmed mixing bowl, dissolve the yeast in the warm water. Let stand 5 minutes until the yeast foams.

2 Stir in the milk, sugar, salt, cardamom, eggs, and 2 cups of the flour; beat until smooth and satiny. Add 2 more cups of flour, beating again until smooth and satiny. Stir in the butter until blended into the batter. Add remaining flour until a dough forms.

3 Sprinkle flour on a clean, dry work surface; turn dough out onto the surface and knead, adding more flour as necessary, to make a smooth, satiny, springy dough.

4 Place ball of dough into a lightly greased bowl; turn dough over to grease the top. Cover with a towel and let rise until doubled, about 1 hour.

5 Turn dough out onto a lightly oiled countertop. Divide into 3 parts. Divide each of the parts into 3, and shape each into a strand about 24 inches long. Braid 3 strands at a time together to make a loaf.

6 Cover baking sheets with parchment paper and place the braided loaves onto the parchment paper. Let rise for about 30 minutes or until puffy but not doubled in size. Meanwhile, preheat oven to 400°F.

7 Brush loaves with beaten egg and sprinkle with almonds and sugar. Bake for about 25 minutes or until a wooden skewer inserted through the loaf comes out clean and dry. Loaves will be light golden brown. Cool on wire rack.

Nutrition Information Per Slice			
Calories	175	Protein (g)	4.5
Fat (g)	3.5	Sodium (mg)	40
Fiber (g)	1	Carbohydrates (g)	30
		Cholesterol (mg)	30

Finnish Rye Bread

—Beatrice Ojakangas

This favored bread of North American Finns is an adaptation of the original sour rye bread. Although you can use stone-ground rye flour in this bread, the very best is made with coarser rye meal. Rye meal is available in whole-foods markets. The authentic bread is shaped into a flat, round loaf about 14 inches in diameter with a hole in the center (somewhat donut-shaped, except flatter). In the western part of Finland, bread baking was done twice a year—hundreds of loaves at a time—in the spring and in the fall. The loaves were strung like beads on poles, then hung across the ceiling of an outdoor storage house especially used for grains. To serve, the bread was cut into wedges, then split like a bun and buttered.

1 Dissolve the yeast in the ¼ cup water in a large, warmed mixing bowl.

2 Add the potato water, brown sugar, and I cup of the rye meal. Let stand 5 minutes until the yeast begins to foam.

3 Add the butter, salt, and bread flour, mixing until a stiff dough forms. Sprinkle the remaining ½ cup rye meal on a board, turn the dough out onto it; cover and let rest for 10 to 15 minutes.

4 Knead until smooth and springy, using rye meal to ease the stickiness. The dough may not take all of the flour. Place dough into a lightly greased bowl; turn dough over to grease the top; cover and let rise for 1 hour or until doubled.

5 Punch down and shape into a round loaf, and place on a lightly greased baking pan. *Or* press the loaf out onto a greased cookie sheet to make a round loaf, 14 inches in diameter and about ¾-inch thick. With fingers poke a hole in the center of the loaf; then gently stretch the hole until it measures about 3 inches in diameter.

6 Let rise again until almost doubled, about 45 minutes. Meanwhile, preheat the oven to 375°F. Prick loaf (both shapes) all over with a fork. Bake loaf for 45 to 55 minutes or until it is crusty and sounds hollow when tapped. Brush with butter while hot.

Makes 1 loaf

1 package (1 T) active dry yeast

¼ cup warm water (105°F to 115°F)

1 cup warm potato water (saved from boiling potatoes) or plain water

1 T brown sugar

1 ½ cups rye meal or stone-ground rye flour

1 T melted butter

½ tsp salt

2 cups bread flour

Finnish Rye Bread *(cont.)*

Nutrition Information Per Slice

Calories	155	Protein (g)	4.5
Fat (g)	1.5	Sodium (mg)	100
Fiber (g)	2.5	Carbohydrates (g)	30
		Cholesterol (mg)	5

Citrus Berry Parfait

—*Anne Patterson*

Serves 4

1 In large bowl of food processor, sprinkle gelatin over lemon juice and lemon peel. Let dissolve for 5 minutes.

2 In small saucepan, heat orange juice to simmer. Pour into food processor. Cover bowl of food processor tightly and blend liquids with dissolved gelatin.

3 Add drained tofu, sugar, and strawberries. Process until smooth, scraping sides of bowl as needed. Pour ¾ cup of mixture into 4 parfait glasses. Chill for at least 2 hours. At serving time, top with strained vanilla yogurt.

1 package unflavored gelatin

3 T fresh lemon juice

1 tsp grated lemon peel

¼ cup orange juice

One 12.3-oz block silken, light, extra-firm tofu, drained

⅓ cup sugar

1 ½ cups fresh or frozen (thawed) strawberries, with juice

1 ½ cups low-fat vanilla-flavored yogurt, strained*

Strain excess liquid from the yogurt by placing it in cheesecloth, coffee filter, or a double-thickness paper towel. Place over a bowl. Cover and let drain, in refrigerator, while parfaits are setting.

Nutrition Information Per Serving	
Calories 235	Protein (g) 20
Fat (g) 2	Sodium (mg) 155
Fiber (g) 1	Carbohydrates (g) 35
	Cholesterol (mg) 5

Orange Poppy-Seed Biscotti

Makes 3 dozen

—Amanda Cushman

2½ cups flour

½ tsp baking powder

½ tsp salt

3 eggs

1 cup sugar

½ tsp orange extract

2 tsp orange zest

⅓ cup toasted almonds

2 T poppy seeds

1 Heat oven to 325°F. Grease and flour a baking sheet.

2 Combine the flour, baking powder, and salt in a medium bowl.

3 With an electric mixer, beat 2 of the eggs with the sugar, orange extract, and orange zest until thick and lemon-colored, about 7 minutes. Add dry ingredients on low speed. Add almonds and poppy seeds.

4 Divide dough into two pieces and shape each into a 9 × 2½-inch log. Place on a baking sheet 2 inches apart. Beat the last egg and brush over the logs.

5 Bake 40 minutes or until golden.

6 Reduce oven to 275°F. Remove logs and let cool slightly, then slice into ¼-inch slices. Arrange cut-side down on baking sheet and bake for 15 to 20 minutes until toasted. Allow to cool before serving.

Nutrition Information Per Serving (2 cookies)			
Calories	130	Protein (g)	3
Fat (g)	2	Sodium (mg)	80
Fiber (g)	>1	Carbohydrates (g)	25
		Cholesterol (mg)	30

Walnut Cake with Cinnamon Syrup

—Amanda Cushman

Makes 3 dozen diamonds

1 Combine the cinnamon syrup ingredients together in a small saucepan and bring to a boil. Stir to dissolve sugar. Cook about 20 minutes. Remove from heat and cool.

2 Preheat oven to 350°F. Combine the butter and sugar in a medium mixing bowl, and beat until light and fluffy. Add eggs, one at a time, beating constantly. Add dry ingredients. Mix in nuts by hand.

3 Grease a 9 × 13-inch baking dish and pour in batter. Bake about 30 minutes, or until knife comes out clean.

4 Remove the cake from the oven and pour syrup onto cake; spread evenly over the top. Cool to room temperature. Cut into diamond shapes.

Cinnamon syrup:

3 cups water

2 cups sugar

1 cinnamon stick

1 slice lemon

1/4 cup rum

Cake:

1 cup butter

1 cup sugar

6 eggs

1 cup flour

1 cup farina

2 1/2 tsp baking powder

1 tsp cinnamon

1 tsp grated orange zest

1 cup finely chopped walnuts

Nutrition Information Per Serving (2 diamonds)

Calories	325	Protein (g)	4
Fat (g)	13	Sodium (mg)	170
Fiber (g)	>1	Carbohydrates (g)	50
		Cholesterol (mg)	90

Sorbetto di Limone e Basilico
(Lemon and Basil Sorbet)

Makes 4 cups

— *Maxine Clark*

8 lemons

2 oranges

2½ cups water

1¾ cups granulated sugar

24 basil leaves

1 Scrub the fruit in warm, soapy water; rinse and dry. Using a sharp potato peeler, remove the peel from the oranges and lemons without chipping the white pith.

2 Place peels in a medium saucepan. Add the water and sugar. Bring to a boil slowly, and boil rapidly for 3 to 4 minutes to reduce slightly the amount of liquid.

3 Remove from the heat, and allow to cool. When cool, strain into a bowl.

4 Meanwhile, squeeze the lemons and oranges; strain, and add juice to the syrup. Tear basil leaves into very small pieces and add to the juice mixture. Chill overnight.

5 Pour liquid into an ice cream maker and let churn for 10 to 15 minutes or until the sorbet is firm enough to serve. To store, quickly scrape sorbet into plastic freezer containers, taking care to mix the basil leaves evenly throughout. Cover with waxed paper and a lid. Label and freeze. Allow 10 to 15 minutes in the refrigerator to soften sufficiently before serving.

Nutrition Information Per Serving (½ cup)	
Calories 190	Protein (g) 5
Fat (g) . . . . >1	Sodium (mg) 1
Fiber (g) . . . . >1	Carbohydrates (g) 50
	Cholesterol (mg) 0

Sorbetto al Cioccolato (Chocolate Sorbet)

—*Maxine Clark*

Makes 4 cups

1 Mix water, both sugars, and cocoa in a saucepan. Bring slowly to a boil, and cook for 4 to 5 minutes, whisking until the sugar dissolves. Reduce the heat and simmer for 3 minutes.

2 Remove from the heat and stir in the chocolate, vanilla, and espresso powder until melted and dissolved. Cool over ice, or allow to cool and chill in the refrigerator. Churn in ice cream maker until frozen.

2½ cups water

¾ cup packed dark brown sugar

½ cup granulated sugar

⅔ cup unsweetened cocoa powder

1 oz bittersweet chocolate, finely chopped

2½ tsp vanilla

1 tsp instant espresso coffee powder

Nutrition Information Per Serving (½ Cup)

Calories 115	Protein (g) 2
Fat (g) 3	Sodium (mg) 5
Fiber (g) . . . . >1	Carbohydrates (g) 25
	Cholesterol (mg) 0

Semi-Freddo di Ricotta al Caffè

Serves 6 to 8

—Maxine Clark

12 oz part-skim ricotta cheese at room temperature

12 oz mascarpone at room temperature (available at specialty food markets)

1 T rum

3 T Tia Maria or other coffee liqueur

1 T vanilla

2 T espresso grounds

Powdered sugar, to taste

A semi-freddo is a dessert that is half frozen to give it a slightly thickened, creamy texture. Ricotta and mascarpone are sweetened, laced with rum and Tia Maria, and flavored with finely ground espresso. The espresso gives an interesting texture. Spooned into white demitasse cups, this is a delightfully rich dessert.

1 Beat the ricotta and mascarpone together in a bowl, using a wooden spoon. (Do not attempt to do this in a food processor or the mixture will become too runny.)

2 Beat in the rum, Tia Maria, vanilla, and espresso. Add powdered sugar to taste. Carefully spoon into demitasse cups or small ramekins, piling the mixture high.

3 Place in the freezer for 2 hours. Transfer to the refrigerator 30 minutes before serving to soften slightly. The dessert should be only just barely frozen or very chilled when served.

4 Just before serving, top each portion with a spoonful of whipped cream and a sprinkling of cocoa. Set on saucers and serve immediately, with squares of bitter chocolate.

Variations: Before freezing, fold in 2 oz toasted chopped hazelnuts and/or 4 oz grated dark bitter chocolate.

Nutrition Information Per ½ Cup

Calories 300	Protein (g) 7	
Fat (g) 23	Sodium (mg) 110	
Fiber (g) 0	Carbohydrates (g) 10	
	Cholesterol (mg) 70	

Global Eating for a Crowd

Global eating is more than a healthy eating philosophy. It's a great way to make your next dinner party even more enjoyable. Parties are an ideal opportunity to introduce new and interesting conversation-starter foods. Why not make your next party an international mix of appetizers, entrées, side dishes, and desserts? When the occasion calls for something special, try the following global recipes.

Appetizers
Dolmádas (stuffed grape leaves), page 152.
Crostini with Chèvre and Tomato Garnish, page 153.
Tsatsíki Sauce with Pita Bread, page 154.
Caponata, page 161.

First Courses
Hot-and-Sour Soup, page 147.
Mediterranean Tabouleh Salad with Parsley and Mint, page 191.
Vegetarian Sushi Rolls, page 187.
Seafood Soup with Rouille, page 206.
Goat Cheese and Black Olive Timbales with Baby Greens, page 192.
Curry Corn Bisque, page 149.

Entrées
Chicken Fried Rice, page 165.
Chicken with Cashews in Hoisin Sauce, page 168.
Sautéed Chicken Breasts with Roasted Garlic Sauce, page 176.
Vegetable Lo Mein, page 181.
Rolled Beef with Vegetables, page 219.
Stuffed Tofu Pasta Shells with Marinara Sauce, page 188.
Provençal Sea Bass, page 203.
Coriander-Crusted Tuna with Parsley Dressing, page 204.
Mediterranean Roast Leg of Lamb, page 223.
Swedish Cheese-Stuffed Chicken Breasts, page 177.
White Onion Pizza, page 195.

Side Dishes
Mediterranean Rice Pilaf, page 183.
Mediterranean Artichoke Hearts and White Bean Stew, page 189.

Desserts

Appendix: The North American Diet at a Glance

A chicken in every pot and a car in every garage.

—Herbert Hoover's 1928 winning presidential campaign slogan, which defined the American Dream.

North America is the land of plenty—where restaurants commonly serve 1,000-calorie meals sans the appetizer and dessert, where supermarket shelves are filled to capacity seven days a week. Where casual-dining restaurants work hard to provide sizeable meals at a fair price, along with the lost sense of family our mobile society has relinquished for its freedom. Yet, perhaps as a result of this superabundance and our willingness to embrace it, the long-term health of many North Americans could be in jeopardy. Consider our track record:

- According to the USDA National Health and Nutrition Examination Survey (NHANES III), 33 percent of U.S. residents are overweight. That's up 8 percent since 1990. At the rate we're going, it's predicted that 100 percent of adults in the United States will be overweight by the year 2030.

- Nearly 8 million cases of diabetes were diagnosed in the United States in 1993, a prevalence that was more than three times that of 1958.

- Nearly 1 in 4 children in the United States is obese, and obese children are more likely to become obese adults. Studies suggest that childhood obesity has triggered an alarming health trend: the pointed increase in the number of children with Type 2 diabetes, a disease once considered to occur mostly in middle age or later.

- Over 50 percent of U.S. adults have a blood cholesterol level over 200, which is medically classified as "borderline-high." About 20 percent of U.S. adults measure "high" cholesterol levels of 240 or higher, without a relatively solid level of "good" cholesterol to protect them. Statistics show that merely by living in the United States, for example, you're at greater risk of dying from heart disease than are the residents of at least sixteen other countries.

• From 1970 to 1990, the U.S. death rate from cancer increased by 7 percent. Because the United States is growing older as a nation, it's predicted that there will be more cases of cancer and cancer deaths, not fewer, unless there is widespread improvement in national health habits.

The good news? The health picture in North America isn't entirely bleak. Life expectancy has reached an all-time high, according to the World Health Organization. Many North American men, for example, can expect to live to age 72; women, to age 79. Furthermore, over the last few decades, deaths from cardiovascular disease in the United States have dropped 50 percent, states the American Heart Association, thanks to better treatments for hypertension, a decline in cigarette smoking among adults, and increased knowledge about heart disease and its risk factors.

What You Eat Can Affect Your Health. On the flip side, what you eat can also do you in. Just as life in general can be hazardous, so too can eating. Chronic diseases can take years to manifest themselves. And during that time, countless bodily reactions can occur that can affect your long-term health both positively and negatively. Metabolism, for example, can contribute to your own demise when free radicals (oxygen molecules that are by-products of the metabolism process that circulate through your bloodstream) attack cells and damage DNA, potentially paving the way for the onset of disease. Meanwhile, other foods such as fruits and vegetables have been hailed as disease fighters, short-circuiting these and other destructive body processes.

Trouble is, we may not be doing enough to aid the "good side" in our own internal battles. When it comes to food selection, a study published in the *Journal of the American Dietetic Association* reported that taste is the most important influence on American food choices, followed by cost. Existing epidemiological evidence suggests that many individuals in North America are undermining their health and their longevity by settling for a diet that's quite tasty yet quite suboptimal.

But take heart. It's not entirely your fault. North America, after all, is a minefield of unhealthy eating opportunities. Fast-food restaurants serving supersized orders of high-fat (but quite appetizing) foods crowd city streets and highways, airports and train stations, shopping malls, even gas stations. Vending machines peddling high-sugar and high-fat snacks (the two almost always come together in snack foods) litter office lunchrooms and coffee stations. Food vendors selling Häagen-Dazs ice cream comb New York City theater aisles during intermissions of off-Broadway plays; you don't even need to leave your seat. Snack carts serving stress relief in the form of packaged pastries, candy, and soda make the rounds daily in companies and corporations.

What's more, the mere whiff of food such as that burger-and-french-fry aroma, which is deliberately piped out onto the sidewalks and walkways of North America through well-placed ventilation, can coax you to eat. So can the mere sight of a strategically planted vending machine. All it takes is a pleasing bouquet or a ten-second glimpse of something glamorous and appetizing, which almost always happens to be high in fat and frequently high in sugar.

A Toxic Environment. Other forces working against the best health interests of you and your family include the car, the remote control, the elevator, the garage door opener, the television, and the computer, which is speedily breeding a new generation of "mouse potatoes." All these forces limit the amount of physical activity we get regularly. Kelly D. Brownell, Ph.D., professor of psychology, epidemiology, and public health at Yale University in New Haven, Connecticut, has gone so far as to dub America a "toxic environment," one that makes eating and *not* exercising easy.

Of course, we can't turn back the clock, nor would we necessarily want to. Would you—or anyone—be willing to use a hand-cranked washing machine or produce your own bread, starting with growing and harvesting your own wheat? Clearly, there are more important ways to spend your time. But experts tell us we would be much better off if walking, taking the stairs instead of the elevator, or biking instead of using the car locally—any form of exercise—were a much bigger part of daily life. According to reports of the surgeon general, more than 60 percent of U.S. adults don't engage in the recommended amount of physical activity of just thirty minutes of moderate activity five or more days of the week. Roughly 25 percent of U.S. adults aren't active at all. According to the Centers for Disease Control and Prevention, at least 200,000 deaths each year from heart disease, cancer, and diabetes could be prevented if those afflicted had not stayed sedentary.

Our Food Past. The "toxic" phenomenon is not exclusive to modern North American life. Like the quiet fortitude of an active volcano, it has been gradually building. Even as far back as the early 1900s, after farming methods became more industrialized, many North Americans ate more than necessary, a factor that was typically related to where they came from originally. "First-generation immigrants were especially focused on food, since food scarcity often had been the prime motivation for their immigration to America in the first place. Generally, diet contained much more meat than was necessary for adequate protein intake, and certainly more meat than these people had been accustomed to eating back in their native lands," writes Elaine N. McIntosh, Ph.D., R.D., in *American Food Habits in Historical Perspective.* The relatively low cost and the abundance of meat in this country, especially succulent fatty meat, made meat especially attractive.

During the 1920s, convenience foods such as breakfast cereals, canned goods, and other prepared foods came on the scene. During this era, the "core" eating pattern of America emerged, which loosely remains the custom today: a citrus fruit or beverage for breakfast, along with cereal or eggs and toast; a modest lunch that includes a sandwich, soup, or salad; and meat as the focal point of dinner, with potato and vegetable side dishes and a simple dessert.

Later, through the depression of the 1930s and World Wars I and II, food production became increasingly mechanized for many North Americans, and our cornucopia continued to runneth over. By the 1960s, meat dominated meals more than ever. At that time, however, a counterculture movement toward vegetarianism began to take hold as health professionals became concerned about the growing prevalence of diet-related chronic diseases and conditions. But then as now, only a small minority of North Americans took part in this change.

Today, despite the plethora in the nation's supermarkets—or perhaps because of it—only 17 percent of North Americans on a given day, meet the U.S. Public Health Service dietary recommendation for fruits, and only 26 percent meet the dietary recommendation for milk products. The government reports that the diet of most people (71 percent) "needs improvement."

References

1. Making Your Diet Go Global

Dietary Guidelines for Americans: For more information, see http://www.usda.gov.

2. The Mediterranean: Olive Oil and Longevity

The healthfulness of the Mediterranean diet—then and now: Antonia Trichopoulou, M.D., and Pagona Lagiou, M.D., *Nutrition Reviews,* November 1997, vol. 55, no. 11, pp. 383–389.

Fat consumption in the U.S.: *Nutrition Insights,* a publication of the USDA Center for Nutrition Policy and Promotion, April 1998.

Meat imports to Greece: E. Helsing, "Trends in fat consumption in Europe and their influence on the Mediterranean diet," *European Journal of Clinical Nutrition,* 1993, vol. 47, Suppl. 1, S4–S12.

Fat intake in present-day Greece: Antonia Trichopoulou, M.D., and Pagona Lagiou, M.D., *Nutrition Reviews,* November 1997, vol. 55, no. 11, pp. 383–389.

Fat intake in present-day southern Italy: Anna Ferro-Luzzi and Francesco Branca, "Mediterranean diet, Italian-style: Prototype of a healthy diet," *American Journal of Clinical Nutrition,* 1995, vol. 61, Suppl. pp. 1338S–1345S.

Percentage of saturated fat in the southern Italian diet: Andrea Bonanome, M.D., Dept. of Internal Medicine, University of Padua, Italy.

Fatal cardiovascular death rates in the Mediterranean: World Health Organization and the American Heart Association. http:www.americanheart.org/Scientific/HSStats98/03cardio.html.

Cancer incidence rates for the Mediterranean: J. Parkin Ferlay, D.M., and P. Pisani, International Agency for Research on Cancer, World Health Organization, *GLOBOCAN 1: Cancer Incidence and Mortality Worldwide in 1990.*

Life expectancy in the Mediterranean: World Health Organization, http://www.who.int/whosis/hfa/countries.

Life expectancy in Spain: *The Lancet,* November 14, 1998, p. 1610(1).

Phenolic antioxidants in olive oil: F. Visiloi, G. Bellomo, et al., "Free radical–scavenging properties of olive oil polyphenols," *Biochemical and Biophysical Research Communications,* June 9, 1998, vol. 1, no. 247, pp. 60–64.

Olive oil imports to the U.S.: U.S. Department of Commerce and the International Olive Oil Council, Madrid.

Health hazards of overweight: "Food, nutrition and the prevention of cancer: A global perspective, 1997," World Cancer Research Fund/American Institute for Cancer Research.

Heart-healthy aspects of the Mediterranean diet: M. de Lorgeril, S. Renaud, et al., "Mediterranean alpha-linolenic acid-rich diet in secondary prevention of coronary heart disease," *The Lancet*, June 11, 1994, vol. 343, no. 8911, pp. 1454–1459.

Cancer-protective aspects of the Mediterranean diet: M. de Lorgeril, P. Salen, et al., "Mediterranean dietary pattern in a randomized trial: prolonged survival and possible reduced cancer rate," *Archives of Internal Medicine*, June 8, 1998, vol. 158, pp. 1181–1187.

Fruit and vegetable consumption in southern Italy: Anna Ferro-Luzzi and Francesco Branca, "Mediterranean diet, Italian-style: Prototype of a healthy diet," *American Journal of Clinical Nutrition*, 1995, vol. 61, Suppl. pp. 1338S–1345S.

Fitness trends in Italy: "World beat: Fitness trends from around the world," IDEA, http://www.ideafit.com/worldbeat.htm.

Cancer incidence among French men: R. J. Black, et al., *EUCAN90* (IARC 1996), 1997, vol. 33, no. 7, pp. 1075–1107.

Trends in smoking in Spain and Italy: A. J. Sasco, "Smoking and social class in France 1974–1991," *Bulletin Cancer*, May 1994, vol. 81, no. 5, pp. 355–359.

3. China: Ancient Nutrition Secrets

History of Chinese food and other cuisine in America: John Mariani, *America Eats Out*, William Morrow, 1991.

Incidence rates of chronic disease in China: *Cancer Facts & Figures–1998*, American Cancer Society, Surveillance Research, 1998. Data source: World Health Organization, 1996.

Diabetes statistics in China: *Diabetes in America*, 2d ed., National Institutes of Health, National Institute of Diabetes and Digestive and Kidney Diseases, NIH Publication no. 95-1468, 1995, p. 664.

Cancer statistics in the U.S.: *Cancer* 1998; vol. 83, pp. 1278–1281, 1425–1432.

How the traditional Chinese diet is becoming more westernized: B. M. Popkin and G. Keyou, The nutrition transition in China: A cross-sectional analysis, *European Journal of Clinical Nutrition*, 1993, vol. 47, pp. 333–346.

Little Emperors/Empresses: Yunxiang Yan, "McDonald's in Beijing: The Localization of Americana." In *Golden Arches East: McDonald's in East Asia*, edited by James L. Watson, Stanford University Press, 1997.

4. France: The Good Life Savored

Fat in the French diet: Adam Drewnowski, Ph.D., and Susan Henderson Ahlstrom, M.S., R.D., et al., "Diet quality and dietary diversity in France: Implications for the French Paradox," *Journal of the American Dietetic Association*, July 1996, vol. 96, no. 7, pp. 663–669.

Heart disease rates in France: See American Heart Association, Cardiovascular Diseases, http://www.americanheart.org/Scientific/Hsstats98/03cardio.html.

Cancer statistics—U.S. and France: R. J. Black, et al., The International Agency for Research on Cancer, European Network of Cancer Registries, "Cancer in the European Union in 1990," *EUCAN90* (IARC 1996), *European Journal of Cancer*, 1997, vol. 33, no. 7, pp. 1075–1107.

Longevity, France and U.S.—See World Health Organization, http://www.int/whosis/hfa/countries.

Centenarians in France: World Health Organization 1998, *The World Health Report 1998—Life in the 21st Century: A Vision for All.*

Alcohol and stroke prevention: *The Journal of the American Medical Association*, 1999, vol. 281, pp. 53–60.

Alcohol and cardiovascular disease: Michael J. Thun, M.D., Richard Peto, F. R. S., et al., "Alcohol consumption and mortality among middle-aged and elderly U.S. adults," *The New England Journal of Medicine*, December 11, 1997, vol. 337, no. 24, pp. 1705–1714.

Snacking and total food consumption: A. Basdevant, C. Craplet, et al., *Appetite*, August 1993, vol. 21, no. 1, pp. 17–23.

Dietary diversity in France: Adam Drewnowski, Ph.D., Susan Henderson Ahlstrom, M.S., R.D., et al., "Diet quality and dietary diversity in France: Implications for the French Paradox," *Journal of the American Dietetic Association*, July 1996, vol. 96, no. 7, pp. 663–669.

U.S. food consumption: See USDA, "Data Used to Calculate the Healthy Eating Index," http://www.nal.usda.gov/fnic/HEI/tab6.html.

Fruit and vegetable consumption in France and Finland: S. M. Artaud-Wild, S. L. Connor, et al., "Plant foods protect the French," *Circulation*, December 1993, vol. 88, no. 6, pp. 2771–2779.

5. Japan: East Embracing West Beautifully and Healthfully

McDonald's locations in foreign lands: McDonald's website at http://www.mcdonalds.com.

Fat consumption statistics in America: Third National Health and Nutrition Examination Survey (NHANES III), 1988–1994.

Heart disease incidence rates—the U.S. and other countries: American Heart Association, *1998 Heart and Stroke Statistical Update.* Dallas, Texas: American Heart Association, 1998.

Breast cancer incidence rates: American Cancer Society, Inc., Cancer Facts & Figures—1998; Abridged Life Tables for Japan, 1995.

Diabetes in the U.S. and other countries: *Diabetes in America*, 2d ed., National Institutes of Health, NIH Publication no. 95-1468, 1995.

Cancer statistics in Japan: National Cancer Institute, D. M. Parkin, C. S. Muir, S. L. Whelan, Y. T. Gao, J. Ferlay, et al., *Cancer Incidence in Five Continents*, vol. VI. IARC Scientific Publication No. 120. World Health Organization, International Agency on Cancer, Lyon, France, 1992.

Life expectancy in Japan: The Japanese Ministry of Health at http://www.mhwgo.jp/english/database/lifetbl/part2.html.

Food consumption information (Japan): National Nutrition Survey conducted by the Ministry of Health and Welfare, http://wwwinfo.ncc.go.jp.

Fish consumption statistics: National Fisheries Institute, USA.

Fish consumption and the 30-year risk of fatal myocardial infarction, M. L. Daviglus, J. Stamler, et al., *The New England Journal of Medicine*, April 10, 1997, vol. 336, no. 15, pp. 1046–1053.

Diabetes in Japan: *Diabetes in America*, 2d ed., National Institutes of Health, NIH Publication no. 95-1468, 1995.

Diabetes incidence and Japanese schoolchildren: *Clinical Pediatrics*, February 1998, vol. 37, no. 2, pp. 111(5).

6. Scandinavia: The Benefits of Dairy and Grains

Heart disease statistics in Finland: P. Pietinen, E. Vartiainen, et al., "Changes in the diet in Finland from 1972 to 1992: Impact on coronary heart disease risk," *Preventive Medicine,* vol. 25, no. 3, pp. 243–250, May–June 1996.

Heart disease statistics in Norway: *Food, Nutrition and the Prevention of Cancer: A Global Perspective,* World Cancer Fund in Association with the American Institute for Cancer Research, 1997.

Coffee consumption in Finland: Terryl J. Hartman, Joseph A. Tangrea, et al., "Tea and coffee consumption and risk of colon and rectal cancer in middle-aged Finnish men, *Nutrition and Cancer,* vol. 31, no. 1, pp. 41–48, 1998.

Fiber and heart disease: D. R. Jacobs Jr, K. A. Meyer, et al., "Whole-grain intake may reduce the risk of ischemic heart disease death in postmenopausal women: The Iowa Women's Health Study," *American Journal of Clinical Nutrition,* vol. 68, no. 2, pp. 248–257, August 1998.

Rye bread consumption and heart disease: P. Pietinen, E. B. Rimm, et al., "Intake of dietary fiber and risk of coronary heart disease in a cohort of Finnish men," *Circulation,* vol. 94, no. 11, pp. 2720–2721, December 7, 1996.

Healthy food perceptions in Denmark: Lars Ovesen, "National policy: Denmark," *Implementing Dietary Guidelines for Healthy Eating,* edited by Verner Wheelock, Blackie A & P, an imprint of Chapman & Hall, London, 1997.

Life expectancy in Denmark: *Ibid.*

Fat content of the Finnish diet: P. Pietinen, E. Vartiainen, et al., "Changes in the diet in Finland from 1972 to 1992: Impact on coronary heart disease risk," *Preventive Medicine,* vol. 25, no. 3, pp. 243–250, May–June 1996.

7. Western Africa: Foods for Cancer Protection

Cancer incidence in Africa: D. M. Parkin, C. S. Muir, S. L. Whelan, Y. T. Gao, J. Ferlay, and J. Powell, *Cancer Incidence in Five Continents,* vol. VI. IARC Scientific Publication no. 120. World Health Organization, International Agency for Research on Cancer, Lyon, France, 1992.

National Cancer Institute: http://rex.nci.nih.gov/ NCI_Pub_Interface/raterisk/rates27.html. *International Range of Cancer Incidence for Selected Sites of Cancer Around 1985,* Females.
http://rex.nci.nih.gov/NCI_Pub_Interface/ raterisk/rates25.html, *International Range of Cancer Incidence for Selected Sites of Cancer Around 1985,* Males.

The cassava: *Fighting hunger with cassava: A gift of 22 recipes from the rural women of Bogso,* African Action on AIDS, The United Nations, NY.

Hypertension rates in The Gambia: M. A. van der Sande, R. Bailey, H. Faal, W. A. Banya, P. Dolin, O. A. Nyan, S. M. Cessay, G. E. Walraven, et al., Nationwide prevalence study of hypertension and related noncommunicable diseases in The Gambia, *Tropical Medicine and International Health,* vol. 2, no. 11, pp. 1039–1048, November 1997.

Economic statistics, demographic information and religious customs, The Gambia: http:// www.odci.gov/cia/publicatioins/factbook/ ga.html.

Peanuts and weight loss: T. A. Pearson, J. P. Kirwan, D. Maddox, V. Fishell, V. Juturu, P. M. Kris-Etherton, *Weight loss and weight maintenance: Effects of high MUFA vs. low-fat diets on plasma lipids and lipoproteins.* The Pennsylvania State University, University of Rochester. Presentation, Experimental Biology '99, April 19, 1999.
K. McManus, L. Antinoro, and F. M. Sacks, *Weight reduction: A comparison of a high unsaturated fat diet with nuts versus a low-fat diet.* Harvard School of Public Health, Harvard Medical School. Presentation, Experimental Biology '99, April 19, 1999.

Peanuts and resveratrol: T. H. Sanders and R. W. McMichael, *Occurrence of resveratrol in edible peanuts.* Presentation, American Oil Chemists Society, Las Vegas, Nevada, 1998.

Peanuts and phytoesterols: A. D. Awad, K. Chan, A. Downie, and C. S. Fink, *Anticancer properties.* University at Buffalo, State University of New York. Presentation, Experimental Biology '99, April 19, 1999.

8. The Gobal Eating Menu Plan for Weight Maintenance or Weight Loss

Exercise habits of the French: Susan Hermann Loomis, "The French are getting fatter," *The New York Times,* September 9, 1998.

Appendix

Overweight in America: Calorie Control Council National Consumer Survey, 1998.

Estimate of overweight Americans by 2030: John Foreyt and Ken Goodrick, "The ultimate triumph of obesity," *The Lancet,* vol. 346, pp. 134–135, July 15, 1995.

Diabetes incidence: *Diabetes in America,* 2d ed., National Institutes of Health, National Institutes of Diabetes and Digestive and Kidney Diseases, 1995.

Heart disease incidence in America and other countries: American Heart Association, 1998.

American consumer food choices: *Journal of the American Dietetic Association,* October 1998, vol. 10, pp. 1118–1126.

America as a "toxic environment": *Nutrition Action Health Letter,* Center for the Science in the Public Interest, July/August 1998.

History of American food habits: *American Food Habits in Historical Perspective,* Elaine N. McIntosh, Ph.D., R.D., Praeger Publishers, 1995.

Percentage of Americans who meet dietary recommendations: "The Diet Quality of Americans," *Nutrition Insights,* a publication of the USDA Center for Nutrition Policy and Promotion, August 1998.

Bon Voyage

B y reading *30 Secrets of the World's Healthiest Cuisines,* we hope you've gained valuable insights into your diet and discovered a whole new world of health information that can help you use your diet to stay healthy for years to come.

In any event, if you'd like to comment on this book, or would like to learn more about how to use international diet secrets to stay healthy, consult our website at http://www.GLOBALEATING.com.

Recipe Contributors

Maxine Clark, the author of seven cookbooks and a food stylist specializing in Italian food, is also a chef at Tasting Places (www.tastingplaces.com), a cooking school that offers a series of weeklong cooking classes in locations throughout Italy and Thailand.

Amanda Cushman is a cooking teacher at Peter Kump's School of Culinary Arts in New York City. She is also a regular contributor to *Vegetarian Times* and *Food & Wine*, and operates her own catering business in Manhattan.

Hope Farrell of Riverside, Connecticut, has been testing and developing recipes for twenty years for various clients, including Robot-Coupe, Cuisinart, Ragu Foods, Media Projects, *Woman's World*, *Reader's Digest* Creative Cooking Club, and *Woman's Day Cookbook*.

Francine Fielding, a recipe tester and recipe developer, lives in Stamford, Connecticut.

Kiyoko Konishi, the owner of Konishi Japanese Cooking in Tokyo, is the author of *Japanese Cooking for Health and Fitness* and *Entertaining with a Japanese Flavor*.

Lynn Kutner is a caterer and cooking instructor in New York City, and is the author of *Bountiful Bread* and *A Pocketful of Pies*. Since the early 1970s, she has also been spending summers with her family in the south of France.

Beatrice Ojakangas is a longtime cookbook author of Finnish descent, whose latest cookbooks include *Whole-Grains by Hand and by Machine* and *The Great Scandinavian Baking Book*.

Anne Patterson is a registered dietitian in Farmington, Illinois, and a consultant to the soy foods industry.

Birgitta Rasmusson is a test-kitchen manager at ICA, a publishing house in Stockholm.

Nikki Rose is a Greek American and a graduate of the Culinary Institute of America. She is currently director of the Washington, D.C.–based World Culinary Arts, an organization that educates American chefs on the food ways of Greece.

Lan Tan is the proprietor of Lan Tan's Chinese Cooking School in Durham, North Carolina.

Francis Trzeciak is the chef and owner of Provence, which offers a little bit of the south of France in Haverford, Pennsylvania. He was born and reared in France, where he studied to be a chef.

Index

About the Authors

Steven Jonas, M.D., M.P.H., M.S., professor of preventive medicine at the State University of New York at Stony Brook, has written eight books of his own and edited/co-authored another ten, on personal health promotion, health policy, and national politics. He has also published more than a hundred professional articles and book reviews, and numerous popular articles on the same health-related subjects. He is editor of the Springer Publishing Company *Series on Medical Education,* an associate editor of *Preventive Medicine,* and a member of the editorial boards of several other professional journals in health promotion/disease prevention. A Fellow of the American College of Preventive Medicine, the New York Academy of Medicine, and the American Public Health Association, Steven Jonas is also a longtime triathlete and a certified professional ski instructor.

Sandra J. Gordon is a freelance health and nutrition writer in Weston, Connecticut. Her articles have appeared in many national publications, including *Fitness, Parents, New Age, Shape, Family Circle, Vitality, Redbook, Mademoiselle,* and *Woman's Day.*